Collaboration and Transition in Initial Teacher Training

**EDITED BY MARGARET WILKIN
AND DEREK SANKEY**

**KOGAN
PAGE**

London • Philadelphia

First published in 1994

Kogan Page Limited
120 Pentonville Road
London N1 9JN

British Library Cataloguing in Publication Data

A CIP record for this book is available from the British Library.

ISBN 0 7494 1107 4

Typeset by Saxon Graphics Ltd, Derby
Printed and bound in Great Britain by Biddles Ltd, Guildford and King's Lynn

Contents

Notes on Contributors

Terry Allsop is a lecturer at the Department of Educational Studies, University of Oxford. For four years he has been Course Tutor for the Internship Scheme.

Eric Bolton is Professor of Teacher Education at the Institute of Education, University of London. He was formerly the Senior Chief Inspector in HM Inspectorate.

Judith Dormer is a teacher in the maths department at Exmouth Community College. She has mentored an articled teacher and students on the University of Exeter pilot school-based scheme.

Anne Evans is Deputy Head and Professional Tutor at Melbourn Village College, Cambridgeshire. She contributed to the planning of the current PGCE secondary course at the Faculty of Education, University of Cambridge and also to the guidelines for induction.

Donald McIntyre is Reader in Educational Studies in the Department of Educational Studies, University of Oxford.

Terence McLaughlin is a lecturer in the Department of Education, University of Cambridge. He is a link lecturer on the University of Cambridge PGCE Course.

David McNamara is Professor of Primary Education, University of Hull. He is Director of the Focused Mentoring for the National Curriculum Project funded by the Paul Hamlyn Foundation.

Rob Moore is a senior lecturer in sociology at Homerton College, Cambridge.

Richard Pring is Director of the Department of Educational Studies, University of Oxford. He was previously Professor and Dean of Education, University of Exeter.

Anne Proctor is Head of Junior Programmes at Edge Hill College of Higher Education. She is closely involved in mentor training programmes.

Geoff Rhodes is Professional Tutor at Larkmead School, Abingdon. He was a member of the Internship Development Group.

Derek Sankey is the Senior Tutor for Initial Teacher Training at the Institute of Education, University of London.

Sarah Tann is a senior lecturer in education for English at Oxford Brookes University.

William Taylor is the former Chair of the Council for Accreditation of Teacher Education. He is now Visiting Professor in the University of Oxford.

Margaret Wilkin is a research fellow at the Centre for Educational Development Appraisal and Research (CEDAR) at the University of Warwick. Until recently she worked in the area of mentoring at the Department of Education, University of Cambridge.

Introduction

The Political and the Professional Perspectives

Teacher training in the UK is at a watershed. In recent years it has been the object of intensive government intervention, which has been motivated principally by strong ideological conviction but also by the need to limit expenditure in an unfavourable economic climate. It has also been experiencing a slow transformation from within. Since the 1970s, and even earlier in the case of the University of Sussex, the relationship between the training institutions and their associate schools has been moving towards one of 'partnership', a term which has come to exemplify a shared, equal and complementary responsibility for the preparation of new recruits to the profession. In general this development has been gradual and evolutionary, although more recently it has been given impetus and leadership by individual partnership schemes such as the Internship Scheme at the University of Oxford and the Area-based Scheme at the Institute of Education, University of London.

There is coincidence between the political and the professional players in two respects: (i) the desirability, indeed necessity of basing beginning teachers in the school for substantial periods, in order that they may learn the skills of teaching from those who practise them; (ii) the value placed on the teachers' contribution to training. However, their fundamental reasons for supporting these two principles are in accord with their respective interests and commitments and are therefore dissimilar. In another regard there is profound disagreement between the politicians and the professionals, both lecturers and teachers, engaged in initial training. This disagreement concerns the kinds of knowledge and practices to which beginning teachers should have access in their training programme, and particularly whether they should be encouraged to develop an ability to theorize about their classroom practice and their situation as beginning teachers in a particular social and political era. For both sides, an appropriate preparation for teaching will provide plentiful opportunities for familiarization with and the acquisition of the practical skills of subject teaching and classroom management. But it is the value of the theoretical input to training that is disputed, whether this is theorizing about the teaching of a subject (what might be called practical theorizing) or the type of theorizing which provides insights into the effects on the teaching process of the many social, political and historical parameters within which school is located. For the government, the ideal teacher is competent, or better, skilful as a teacher of a subject in the classroom, is able to assess pupils' progress, manage their learning experiences and maintain order. These aspirations are shared by the teacher training profession. It would be nonsensical for it to be otherwise. But the profession's ideal teacher is, in addition, critically reflective about the process of education and the teacher's role as a practitioner within it. The profession and the government disagree therefore less on the site of training (though this is a question of degree) than on its substance. The two cases represent two fundamentally different perceptions of the aims of teacher training and hence the sort of people we wish our teachers to be.

In order to demonstrate how similar in some respects, but also how profoundly different are the preferred forms of training of the politicians and the professionals, we will look at each in turn, starting with the former. There are two reasons why successive Conservative governments have wished to see the training of teachers become predominantly school-based: a desire to see the quality of training improved, and a commitment to reshaping the institutions of society in accordance with the ideological principles of 'Thatcherism'. These two justifications for intervening in initial training are inextricably interwoven and over time the latter has come to dominate the former.

'Better Schools', a White Paper issued in 1985, linked teacher training and the principles of Thatcherism and was an early indication of the developments that lay ahead. It expressed concern that standards in schools were not as good as they might be and that therefore there was a need to improve the professional effectiveness of teachers. But it also noted that education in schools should promote enterprise, and that higher standards would reinforce government policies to strengthen the economy. Subsequently the government has gone beyond the suggestion that good teaching will promote its ideological ends, thereby implying in rhetoric at least that teachers are to be its indirect 'agents'. Through Circulars 24/89 (DES, 1989) and 9/92 (DfE, 1992) it has transformed the system of training itself. Criteria for approval of initial teacher training courses in Circular 24/89 include the requirements that student teachers should spend a substantial part of the training period in school and that experienced teachers should be involved in the planning and evaluation of courses, the selection of students and the supervision and assessment of students' practical work. In Circular 9/92 these proposals are extended. The Circular addresses schools engaged in training as 'partner schools' and expects them to exercise a joint if not leading responsibility for the planning and management of courses. Partner schools are required to show that they are able to contribute to training, that they have a good staff development record and adequate facilities. By the end of the training period students must have a wide understanding of their subject ('subject knowledge'); they must know how to transmit it ('subject application'); they must be able to maintain order ('class management') and to assess and record pupil progress; and they must have acquired *inter alia* the ability to identify special needs and some understanding of the school as an institution. In Circular 24/89 there was a section headed 'Education and Professional Studies'; in the later circular, there is no such section.

It can be seen that the government has realigned teacher education to a quite remarkable degree. With considerable political audacity it has brought about changes in the structure and practices of training as well as in the distribution of power between tutors and teachers, and in so doing has reversed a situation which in most institutions had existed for decades. In the past, by providing 'teaching practice' places for students, the schools serviced the HEIs. While undoubtedly teachers did undertake some unofficial teaching of students, there was no requirement nor even expectation that they would do so. They had no formal role as trainers, their task being to supervise students who put into practice the teaching methods that they had been taught in the lecture or seminar room. It was quite usual for tutors to visit students every week and for tutors to direct the work of the student within the school, thus extending the influence of the HEI into the school itself. Teachers were usually, though not always, asked to assess student progress, but their views probably carried less weight in the final grade awarded to the student for practical teaching skill than the views of the tutor. To further demonstrate the value that it attributes to school-based training the government has also introduced 'school-led' training schemes, in which professional preparation is located within the school and in which 'ownership' of the student has been removed from the HEI. Included here are teachers training under the Licensed Teacher Scheme or in the new consortia of training schools which are in receipt of direct funding.

These changes can be interpreted politically. In several respects the form that teacher training takes today reflects the ideology of the social market, of Thatcherism. It places training in the hands of the practitioners, it marginalizes theorists, it provides choice, and it encourages individualism. Placing training, though not administration or assessment, largely in the hands of teachers meets two ideological principles. Teachers are the 'producers' of teaching, and in the training process, the 'consumers' are the students. By mediating as it were in this relationship, tutors disrupt the exchange of skills. If training is placed in the hands of the producers of training then this must be the most efficient system. If tutors are removed from the training process, or their influence is minimalized, then teacher-producers have direct access to student-consumers. Furthermore, tutors are theorists and in the doctrine of the social market, it is the practitioners, the doers, who are privileged over theorists. Theorists are perceived as unproductive; their activities failing to result in anything tangible or clearly definable. As Thatcher herself said at the Party Conference of 1988: 'We have the great assurance that our beliefs are not lofty abstractions confined to philosophy lectures. They are the common sense of the people' (Thatcher, 1989).

The current arrangements for the training of students represent the political perspectives of the government in other respects. It is now possible to choose a course of training from a wide range of routes, and choice is the central principle in the philosophy of the market. The would-be teacher can train by attending an HEI and taking a BEd or PGCE course; can train through the Licensed Teacher Scheme; or can go directly into a school and train within a single school. Moreover, students on whatever form of training course are today required to demonstrate 'individualism' to a much higher degree than students of initial training ten or 15 years ago, where individualism is interpreted as the ability to look after one's own interests, to shape one's social environment and to take responsibility for personal achievement. Irrespective of the course they are on, students spend longer periods away from the host HEI. They may receive their training in any of a wide variety of schools each of which will have its own ethos and its own views on how training in school should be undertaken. A student may be the only trainee in the school. Other students in mainstream training may find when they meet up with the fellow students that their experiences differ widely and somehow they have to make sense of these discrepancies and learn how to make the most of their particular situations. In all of these respects, the changes to training which have been enforced through legislation reflect its political doctrines.

Four points should be made concerning the above comments. First, it is important to acknowledge the right of the politicians to their perspective. It is an anticipated political practice – and therefore should come as no surprise – that governing groups will strive to dominate society by restructuring or realigning social institutions in accordance with their ideological principles. By so doing, they extend their influence and hope to persuade the mass of the people of the value of their own views of the world. Second, and this is related to the above, there is no necessary association between central control of social institutions and the commitments, attitudes or values of those who work within them. Disclosures concerning the politicization of teacher training should therefore not be taken to imply any comment on the views or attitudes of either tutors or teachers. Third, a number of the changes that have been introduced by the government – for example placing students in schools for longer periods and agreeing that teachers should have more responsibility for their professional development – were already embryonic characteristics of the training system. They could be found in a limited number of institutions where they were voluntary rather than compulsory arrangements which had been entered into for the professional benefits they were deemed to provide. Finally, and crucially, there is considerable accord between politicians and professionals regarding the importance for both professional and moral reasons of conferring on teachers a much greater responsibility than they have had hitherto for the training of beginning teachers. Teachers have expertise above all in the skills of subject delivery and classroom management and these are the areas in which it is crucial for the student to acquire immediate proficiency.

We can now consider from the perspective of the profession changes that were outlined above. There it was noted that Circular 9/92 had no section on educational or professional studies, and it is difficult to find any reference at all in that document either to theory or to theorizing. This is surely a logical omission as well as a display of ideological petticoats. The task of the teacher (now the mentor) in school-based training is to assist the beginning teacher in the improvement of his or her practice. This will entail reviewing with the student what has been achieved, how a particular practice could be improved, and so on. Such a discussion with the mentor will introduce the student to the 'theory' of that practice, that is the principles on which it is based. All rational, directed and systematic activity is underpinned by theory, although this may be forgotten when activities become well-established, even routine, and are executed without conscious thought. The student in the school is surrounded by theory although much of this theory may be covert. Not only is every current teaching practice underpinned by theory, but particularly today, teachers are confronted with numerous issues that require 'theorizing'. The National Curriculum, league tables and the nature of sex education are examples of such issues. Thus even if teacher training were to take place entirely in schools, this would not commit the student to a theory-less environment as is so often implied. Teachers are experts at practical theorizing and in their mentoring of students this theorizing will be articulated, either explicitly or by implication. Sharing theorizing with the students about their respective forms of practice is at the heart of the mentor's task.

Above, the mentoring role was portrayed as consisting of the management of student learning in support of skill acquisition. This was quite a straightforward representation of what is a highly skilled task and one about which it is easy to imagine theorizing taking place. For example, the mentor may reflect on whether she or he has been overhasty in introducing the student to whole-class teaching, and could improve therefore on the diagnostic skills that mentoring requires. It is 'easy' to imagine theorizing here, not because it is not an important intellectual activity but because the theorizing takes place within a known set of circumstances and within known parameters. In cases like this of practical theorizing, we modify existing practices and in this way hope to improve professional performance. But when, say, the concept of mentoring is investigated in a research project, a whole range of unexpected issues may be disclosed. 'Mentoring' suddenly becomes like a magnet which has attached to it all manner of different perspectives which were invisible until now. This sort of discovery theorizing is concerned less with investigating, developing and improving the known, at least initially, than with using the known as a starting point to investigate the as yet unknown. But once the unknown has become known, then it can be integrated into the known and used for its sophistication. It is this type of theory and theorizing, that which is characterized by the unknown, the surprising, the shock of revelation, which is the characteristic theory of higher education; and it is theorizing of a quite different kind to that of practical theorizing. One is not better than the other. They are of a different order, and both have their uses. 'Practical theorizing' could be said to *improve* the status quo. What may be called 'intellectual theorizing' *changes* the status quo by introducing alternative interpretations of the same reality. (There is of course no suggestion here that practical theorizing is somehow unintellectual). Intellectual theorizing induces a mental jump, a reassessment, a recognition that what has appeared to be stable and complete is on the contrary only one way of understanding a particular social phenomenon.

The disagreement of the professionals with the politicians centres on the minimal role attributed to theory and theorizing (both practical and intellectual) by the latter. If it is mainly, although not exclusively, the task of the mentor to introduce the student to practical theorizing – this is common sense – how necessary is it that the student trainee has access both to the process and content of the sort of theorizing which is here called 'intellectual' and which is so central a component of the culture of higher education? One's response to this question will depend amongst other things upon the status that one attributes to teaching as an occupational activity. If teaching is to be a profession, and if we want our teachers to exercise critical reflection because this quality, conferred by higher education, is valued, then the diminution of the university or college component of the initial training curriculum is to be deeply regretted, more, to be opposed. If training to become a teacher becomes divorced from higher education, then teaching will be placed on a level with those occupations for which an apprenticeship form of induction is considered sufficient. Here the trainee receives tuition and guidance in practice and is introduced to practical theory. But he or she will not have access to the vision that forces a reassessment of things as they are – the reason perhaps for the current exclusion of theory from the curriculum of training.

The Current Scene

The government initiatives outlined above were introduced with characteristic rapidity and forcefulness and their consequences have been profound. The 'simple' requirement that students should spend more time in school and that teachers – now mentors – should not merely supervise them but actually share responsibility for their training, in reality is enormously complex to implement. It raises a whole range of issues of a *practical* nature: about the logistics of student numbers and their allocation to schools, about the redistribution of funding, about the construction of a course which must meet government requirements. It also raises numerous *professional* issues: how can schools be prepared – and prepare themselves – to assume these new responsibilities, and how can training be monitored and the student experience be made comparable across so many sites? Then there are *personal* issues: about the need for both tutors and teachers to adapt to and train for changing roles, about adjustment to realigned relationships of power. And so on. In the centre of these swirling currents of change there is the student, whose needs as a beginning teacher must come first.

The chapters in this book are intended as a commentary on the contemporary scene in initial teacher training, and it is hoped that they will appeal to readers in schools as well as those in training institutions. There are some contributions from teachers, although inevitably at this stage the majority are from those in HEIs. The chapters develop the themes both implicit and articulated in the discussion above. They are not sub-divided into sections as is usually the case in a collection of this sort, but for those who have the stamina, are designed to be read through consecutively. The opening chapter sets the scene and the focus progressively moves into the school. In the centre of the collection there are eight chapters all of which are 'school-focused'. We then move away from the school again with a chapter on the maintenance of quality within the training system as a whole, and the collection ends with a chapter which looks towards the future. The text portrays a system in transition. Excitement at new challenges is evident as is doubt and anxiety. Above all there emerges a strong commitment to the provision of a quality training, through partnership.

The first chapter roots contemporary changes in initial training in the interest taken by both political parties in standards in schools in the 1970s and early 1980s. Concern about the effectiveness of teacher training emerged as a consequence of a growing apprehension about our educational standards relative to those of our international competitors. Subsequently the motivation for government intervention in training shifted from the educational to the cultural. Bolton suggests that the progressive distancing of initial training from higher education which has taken place over recent years, through for example the Licensed Teacher Scheme and the proposed Teacher Training Agency (TTA) represents an agenda which has less to do with training teachers than with the reduction of potential political opposition. In an interesting comparison with the training methods of the last century, he identifies the policies of the government today as an attempt to return teacher training to a quasi-apprenticeship system which is divorced from the radical ideas of higher education. This is also a theme taken up in the next chapter by Moore, who locates recent political initiatives in teacher training within a broadly-based attack on liberalism and the professions. The thread running through this deeply felt chapter is the relationship between theory and practice. Moore suggests that the way in which 'theory' is used by the government is partial and opportunistic. The place and role of theory in training is dismissed, yet the highly theoretical nature of government policy remains unacknowledged. He continues with a discussion on the respective forms of expertise of tutor and teacher. This is not a distinction between theory and practice – for the work of each is both theoretical and practical in turn – but between the production of knowledge and application of knowledge. These have in common and are linked by the 'third practice', that of reflexivity, 'the cultivation of which as a general attitude of mind and an approach to life is what education in the liberal tradition is ultimately all about'.

The next chapter by Allsop takes us into the school. Its concern is the development of a language of partnership, and what the comments of teachers and interns (students) tell us about the operation of a school-based scheme. He concludes that it takes time for the trust and confidence between the partners in training to be reflected in a shared language. He also notes the way in which comments from the school staff disclose the problems and the small irritations which accompany participation in training even in a well-established scheme. However, the remarks of interns suggest an excitement and pride in becoming a teacher and also an appreciation of the way in which they are received by schools.

Chapters 4 and 5 are by professional tutors in two different school-based schemes, and taken together they provide a comprehensive picture of the professional tutor's role. Both writers were members of the planning groups which devised their respective schemes, and their chapters illustrate well the extent to which participation in training by schools necessitates considerable internal changes of both a structural and organizational nature. The focus of the first is the way in which the school now exercises autonomy and discretion in implementing the training curriculum. Basing her account on her own experience, Evans describes four aspects of training which her partnership school now undertakes: induction, day-to-day mentoring, the school-based seminar and 'extended professional experience'. She then moves on to outline some principles which will facilitate the transition to schools of curricular responsibility. Rhodes' chapter, also based on experience in a partnership scheme, presents an additional and alternative view of the professional tutor's task: that of the general management of student learning, including the leadership of mentors and the integration of students into the school; he also discusses the necessity for training to be a whole-school commitment. Historically, politically and professionally these two accounts are interesting. They are powerful and confident in tone, and it is difficult to imagine their having been written even five years ago. Both writers are strongly supportive of maintaining a collaborative partnership with their respective HEIs because of the distinctive contribution to training that each partner can make.

Chapters 6 to 11 are all 'within' the school. McIntyre (Chapter 6) introduces us to the classroom as a learning environment and so provides a valuable context for the two chapters which follow. It begins with a reminder that classrooms are necessarily the principal sites of learning for beginning teachers, but ends with a word of warning: that placing training predominantly in schools is no guarantee of a quality training. He reviews the difficulties faced by students in school when training was in the hands of the HEIs. Then there was a lack of collaboration between tutors and teachers and the student learned to survive, and teachers had neither the authority nor the confidence to engage in training. But if teachers assume responsibility for the professional education of students then their practice in this regard will need to become purposeful and structured. They will need to perceive themselves differently, to become educators of student teachers.

There follow two chapters which complement that of McIntyre. They look at training to teach from the inside, from the perspective of the student. The first by Tann (Chapter 7), is a sensitive account which suggests learning to teach is an anxiety-provoking experience in which the student has to make sense of the respective nuggets of advice of teacher and tutor, and achieve their reconciliation or make choices between them. The teacher (mentor) and the tutor are perceived as having different sorts of advice to offer which are valued for different reasons and at different stages in the beginning teacher's professional development. Questions are raised about the best way to introduce students to the vast array of knowledge that they are now required to demonstrate, and the importance of the teacher being responsive to the variability of student need is stressed.

The second chapter on the student perspective (Chapter 8) is a wide ranging review of the 'determinants' of beginning teachers' practices in the classroom. McNamara finds that the requirements of the National Curriculum heavily constrain the freedom that the primary student teacher can exercise with regard to curriculum choice, but that there are greater opportunities for experimentation in the area of method. The third section of this chapter is perhaps the most interesting because the least expected. It suggests that there is an element of randomness in learning to teach which is rarely acknowledged. It reviews students' perceptions of the various sources of influence on their teaching. 'Although the data should be interpreted with caution', students appear to nominate mentors and tutors in equal proportion, but also nominate other sources (including 'common sense') to a comparable extent. The final section of the chapter warns that learning to teach is considerably more complex than putting 'common sense' into practice. Teacher training should aim to familiarize the student with alternative approaches to the teaching of a subject and encourage a broad perspective on the teacher's role in general.

Having been with the student in the classroom for the previous two chapters as it were, we now move on to discussions between mentor and student on student achievement (Chapters 9 and 10). Chapter 9, by Dormer is an account of an investigation of the role of the mentor which was stimulated by her own experience as a mentor of an Articled Teacher. She concludes that all categories of beginning teachers need both challenge and support in the mentoring relationship, although in varying proportions, if they are to make progress. She devises a tiered model of mentoring based on these dimensions which could be of value in giving direction to induction at different levels within the profession. Chapter 10, which follows, elaborates this model. With the intention of providing examples of tutors' supervisory strategies that mentors might find useful to consider, Proctor selects extracts from tutors' notes to student teachers whom they have observed in the classroom. These notes are then analysed and the range of strategies used highlighted: the use of instruction, the setting up of a dialogue, the encouragement of reflection and so on, as considered appropriate. She then isolates three key areas of supervision and indicates their relevance for mentoring, and by so doing, like Dormer, suggests a way in which mentoring can become a structured and purposeful activity.

Chapter 11, the third which focuses closely on the mentors' role is a detailed account of the process of mentoring. McLaughlin begins his discussion by contrasting an apprenticeship model of training with a 'more adequate professional' model of training. He then critically reviews the concept of reflection on practice, arguing that in any worthwhile form of training, reflection will inevitably raise questions about issues wider than immediate practice. This chapter therefore has important implications for how the mentor's role in encouraging reflection is conceived, since it cannot be limited to consideration of immediate practice, but necessarily must make reference to more general issues. He criticizes the loose manner in which the term is frequently used and concludes by suggesting ways in which the quality of reflective discussion with the student can be enhanced.

'Quality' is the theme of Chapter 12. The movement of training into schools raises very real problems about the monitoring of quality. Taylor reviews the history of quality control in teacher preparation and reminds us that quality requirements will now apply just as much to the school-based elements of training as to those located in the training institutions. How can this be done on such a large scale? The attitudes, practices and procedures on which current mechanisms for monitoring and maintaining quality in the HEIs depend, will have to be extended into schools and a 'quality culture' established. This means that everyone at whatever level who is engaged in the training of beginning teachers should be constantly monitoring and assessing the quality of their work.

The final chapter looks to the future. Pring makes a realistic assessment of the financial implications of maintaining the current system and concludes that it cannot survive in its present form. He reviews the background to the debate on the relationship between theory and practice in training, and highlights the way in which current policy mitigates against the academic respectability of teaching as a profession by removing it from universities and all that they stand for. The future is not entirely bleak however, because the government is unlikely to be able to control training if it is dispersed to schools and teachers themselves see the advantages of retaining the connection with institutions of higher education. There will therefore still be training institutions in the future although these may be greatly reduced in number. Their function will revert to that traditionally associated with universities – research and scholarship – while training in schools becomes institutionalized. The success of training will depend upon combining the distinctive forms of expertise of schools and HEIs.

The chapters in this book portray a profession reorienting itself within a framework of political and professional demands. Necessarily, roles are being redefined and it is appropriate that it is the roles of the staff in school which receive the greater attention at the moment since that is where training is now principally to be located. But the role of the tutor is also changing. That students need and look for the contribution of tutors to their professional understanding emerges in several of the chapters. That contribution is seen by the student as of a certain kind, and as particularly appropriate at a certain stage. If mentors provide the here-and-now guidance for the student in the classroom, tutors are seen as providing access to the wider view derived from research; and there is a suggestion that in future the tutor may become more distant from direct practice, leaving this to the mentor, and become more fully engaged than at present in the pursuit of research.

How should these changes be regarded? Are they a process of evolutionary development spurred on by government perhaps but essentially an outworking of ideas and practices already existing, albeit in embryonic form? Or do they constitute a revolutionary change in the form and content of training, a paradigm shift, when as a result of a perceived crisis, a new order is brought into being, replacing old ways of working and thinking about initial training? Certainly the government would wish to claim the latter. It did perceive a crisis in education and was persuaded that the content and methods of teacher training were partly, even largely to blame. It has imposed through regulation what appears to be a new order in which the balance of time and responsibility has been shifted towards schools and serving teachers. But in so far as all the main elements of this 'revolution' were being introduced by the profession itself, the nature of the change is closer to an evolutionary model where gradual development occasionally receives a more dramatic thrust.

It is important in the highly politicized climate of training today that continuities with the past are recognized. To do so gives a sense of direction in the current maelstrom that is teacher training, and helps to restore to some degree at least a sense of professional autonomy in the face of the control that is currently being exercised. The need for collaboration now and in the future between the two partners of school and training institution was never greater. Currently our concerns must be to provide the best training we can for our students while these transitional upheavals are taking place. Only if schools and training institutions each contribute their expertise to the professional preparation of teachers will teaching remain a profession; but also only if that is the case will that preparation remain professionally adequate.

References

DES (1989) *Initial Teacher Training: Approval of Courses* (Circular 24/89), London: DES.
DfE (1992) *Initial Teacher Training (Secondary Phase)* (Circular 9/92), London: DfE.
Thatcher, M (1989) *Party Conference Speeches 1975–1988*, London: Conservative Political Centre, p 143.

Chapter 1

Transitions in Initial Teacher Training: An Overview

Eric Bolton

In 1976 the then Prime Minister, James Callaghan, made an important speech at Ruskin College, Oxford, about education. His speech was noteworthy for two main reasons. First he raised some particular and quite serious criticisms of our school education system and what went on within it. Second, he indicated that the government intended to take a direct interest in the curriculum, how well it was taught, its relevance, and the standards being achieved. This announcement of direct government involvement was greeted by shock/horror in the education world.

Ten years later, the involvement of government was much more direct and marked, and a Conservative government led by Margaret Thatcher had given its particular gloss and direction to central government's interest in education. Keith Joseph had become the Secretary of State for Education and Science in 1981 and had instigated, among other things, a systematic analysis of the strengths and weaknesses of the English school system. That analysis was completed in 1986 and brought to fruition in the White Paper 'Better Schools'. This White Paper called for standards to be raised at all levels; confirmed the introduction of the GCSE to replace the previous examinations at 16 plus, and pointed out that our greatest failing, in comparison with other similar countries, was that we did not usefully qualify the broad mass of ordinary pupils. To address that problem, and to raise standards, the White Paper called for national agreement about what should be included in the school curriculum and about the standards that should be expected and achieved. In effect, 'Better Schools' laid down the basis for the curriculum and assessment legislation that would follow 18 months or so later in the Education Reform Act (ERA) of Kenneth Baker.

The ERA introduced new reforms intended to create choice and competition, and also an education market that reflected the macro-philosophies of Thatcherite conservatism. It also confirmed in legislation the National Curriculum, and its associated forms of assessment, that had developed out of the long-running, cross-party political debate of the previous decade. Behind both the new curriculum and standards legislation, and the more political acts-of-faith of the education market legislation, lay a shared and common concern to raise standards in education across the board. Consequently, quality, relevance, breadth and depth of study and standards became the key words in the education debate.

Sooner rather than later, any discussion of quality in education brings to the fore questions about the quality and effectiveness of teachers and teaching. In fact, successive governments throughout the 1960s, 70s and 80s sought to influence the education and training of teachers in one way or another, even when, as in the 1960s and early 70s, they were apparently uninterested in questions relating to curriculum, standards, and teaching and learning.

With the advent of the first Thatcher government in 1979, things changed markedly. By the early 1980s, it was clear that the new conservative government was going to take a closer interest in what was taught in schools, and the quality and standards achieved. Initially it focused on the quality of teaching and initial teacher training. In 1983 the then Secretary of State, Joseph, published a White Paper, 'Teacher Quality'. This was quickly followed by Circular 3/84 which established the Council for the Accreditation of Teacher Education (CATE), and set out the ground rules and specific criteria that would have to be satisfied by all initial teacher training courses if they were to be accredited by the Secretary of State to award Qualified Teacher Status (QTS). The general drift of the criteria was to diminish the time spent during training on academic/theoretical study, and to increase the time spent by students in some form of practical teaching. As these reforms began to impinge upon courses, the shape and content of initial teacher training (ITT) courses began to change. In addition, a series of HMI reports on individual teacher training institutions and courses was published, further opening up public discussion about teacher training.

Essentially, this was the nature of government influence on ITT in the run-up to the Education Reform Act of Kenneth Baker in 1988. In effect the government's attention during those years moved from teacher training (though never wholly so) to the school curriculum, and to questions of quality and standards of pupil performance and achievement which necessarily had implications for the relevance and quality of teacher training. The emergence of the National Curriculum, and its related assessment, introduced new and additional requirements for all ITT courses. These had particularly onerous consequences for primary teacher training as the whole weight of the extensive National Curriculum had to be carried by each primary school teacher.

Even though it had paid most attention to schools and serving teachers, it would not be true to say that during that period the government was relaxed about, or contented with, teacher training. Far from it. It frequently revealed its dissatisfaction and that it still harboured suspicions about the motives of teacher trainers; in particular that the trainers took a certain ideological line and worked against the implementation of government education policy. However, most of the time available was taken up by determining the legislation effecting schools. In addition, throughout the early to late 1980s, the economic boom led to acute supply problems in teaching. Consequently, it was not the time to do anything by way of radical reform that might worsen an already difficult situation. In short, in certain areas of the country, and in a good number of specialist subjects, we needed all the teachers we could get. At times like that, questions about entry standards, or indeed about exit standards, while not unimportant, become less pressing.

By the early 1990s the national picture was beginning to change. The boom had clearly ended. Economic recession was the reality of the time and there was a more than adequate supply of bright and capable people coming into teaching. In fact, the signs were of an impending national surplus of primary teachers. There had also been important changes at ministerial level. By 1991, Kenneth Clarke was the Secretary of State, and John Major had replaced Thatcher as the Prime Minister.

For a number of complex reasons, the government's policy intentions began to turn again to the quality of teachers and teaching. Among these was the fact that the implementation of the ERA, and in particular of the assessment regulations, was leading to difficult confrontations with the teachers, not only about curricular content or forms of testing, but also about teaching styles, methodologies and philosophies of educating the young.

Those concerns came to a head around the end of 1990 and the beginning of 1991 when the country entered into one of those periodic scares about standards of literacy and the teaching of reading and writing which we seem to suffer every decade or so. This is not the place to explore why that came about when it did, save to say that it came at a time when the government was under great pressure about many of its education policies and when Major, as an unelected Prime Minister at the time, was trying to establish a distinctive domestic policy prior to an imminent general election. He decided that the issues of basic standards, of the quality of teachers and of teaching styles were vote-winners for a Conservative Prime Minister and ought to be given prominence.

Consequently, the attention given to ITT began to take on a rather different caste under Clarke and Major from that which had applied during the regimens of Joseph and Baker. Some old concerns remained, namely, that teacher-educators and the training courses they ran were ideologically predisposed against the policies of Conservative governments, and were in the control of the soft, progressive left. A related but older belief was reasserted, that the teaching profession generally, and primary teachers in particular, had been seduced away from sound traditional teaching methods into progressive, soft-centred relativism by academic teacher trainers and various assorted gurus. Academic standards had suffered as a consequence. Perhaps even more important was the right-wing conviction that standards of behaviour and morality were also being put at risk by the ideologies that were deemed to dominate much of the teaching in schools, particularly primary schools, and which in the demonology at least, seemed to stem from teacher-training institutions.

The change of direction arising from the re-emergence of those older concerns about teaching and teacher education, and the pressures of an imminent general election, resulted in education becoming a populist issue with back-to-basics as its rallying cry and caused a significant shift in the debate about teacher training. That shift in essence was away from specifics about methodology, content or competence towards more fundamental questions of cultural values. That it is not to say that content, methods and competences disappeared from the national debate about teacher training. On the contrary, they are heavily present, but they are no longer the engine driving the debate. Nor are they in the government's eyes the major justification for further radical changes to ITT. This lies in a fundamental questioning about the kind of people teachers ought to be; about the perceptions of human nature, and of our social institutions, that ought to inform teaching in our schools. In effect the debate about teacher training has become a debate about fundamental values implicit in, and transmitted by, teachers and schools.

In recent times there have been a number of manifestations of this change. In December 1991 the then Secretary of State, Clarke, issued a statement about primary education. It was remarkable for a number of reasons. In particular it led to an enquiry by the chief inspector (HMI) for primary education, Jim Rose. Christopher Woodhead, then the chief executive of the National Curriculum Council, and Robin Alexander of Leeds University were to report to him on primary teaching methods and classroom organization. But at the same time Clarke made it clear that he intended to reform the training of primary school teachers making it more classroom-based, and to transfer more responsibility for training from colleges and universities to the schools themselves. At the time he suggested that 80 per cent of training might be done in and by schools.

The statement went on to explore at some length issues of methodology and organization, and to criticize progressive child-centred philosophies that the Secretary of State saw as being responsible for most, if not all, the weaknesses of primary education in England. The document had no praise for, and much criticism of, the role of higher education in training teachers. The report from the so-called 'Three Wise Men' was produced in record time and it was followed by new regulations for the training of primary school teachers from the Department for Education.

In the event the general election intervened. The Conservative party won; Clarke moved on to higher things and John Patten became the Secretary of State. Following the promise of his predecessor to reform ITT, Patten issued Circular 9/92 which was, rather surprisingly, about the secondary PGCE rather than primary training. The circular required secondary teacher training to be predominantly school-based and, implicitly and explicitly, was cool towards higher education. Much later, in June 1993, a draft circular on the initial training of primary school teachers was issued by the DfE, followed in November 1993 by Circular 14/95, providing the new criteria for primary training courses for September 1996 onwards. As with the new secondary courses, the circular extended the time spent in school and school involvement and required that courses be planned in partnership with participating schools.

The government has continued to chip away at ITT. It has done so through the Articled Teacher Scheme; the Licensed Teacher Scheme; its new consortia proposals by which groups of schools can cluster together and recruit their own students and train them; and through its draft proposal for what came to be called the 'Mums Army'. The intention of that proposal was to enable schools to recruit and train teachers who would not only not need to be graduates on entry to training, but who would not need to be graduate, or graduate equivalent, at completion of training. That small move, now shelved, would have dismantled the only recently achieved all-graduate status of teaching in England and Wales. In September 1993, another set of proposals emerged from the government called, prosaically,

'The Government's Proposals for Initial Teacher Training'. That document moved further towards dismantling the current pattern of ITT by decoupling it more generally from higher education. Significantly for the longer-term shape of ITT, it proposed a new Teacher Training Agency (TTA) to organize, fund and determine the shape and pattern of teacher training in England, and of research and higher degrees in education. In pursuing those particular aims and further extending the notion of school-centred training (SCITT) this proposal continues to weaken the links between QTS and higher education graduate or post-graduate qualifications. In the proposed consortia schemes, higher education no longer has a defined role.

The general drift of government policy is clear: namely to break up the more-or-less monolithic pattern of ITT and to decouple it from higher education. This raises the spectres of some much older debates, such as those of the 1860s. At that time, Battersea College under the influence of Kay-Shuttleworth and the National Society, was providing teacher training based on notions of pastoral simplicity, service and humility. Its concern was largely with character formation and on training teachers for the workhouse schools. Teachers trained in a simple and demanding way would, 'as a result of the laborious and frugal life... go forth into the world humble, industrious and instructed' (Kay-Shuttleworth, 1862). Not too well instructed and certainly non-participants in academic education. The decent, humble poor were trained to educate the deserving poor in ways that would not stir them up too much, or give them too many radical ideas.

In contrast to Battersea, St Mark's College Chelsea, with Derwent Colridge as its first principal, emphasized academic education and upward social mobility. It recruited grammar school boys who followed two years of their own academic studies with Latin as the core. This is echoed in today's BEd requirement that students do at least two years study at higher education level. The students spent a great deal of time in the college chapel participating in high church, Anglo-Catholic services and large numbers entered the church rather than teaching.

A third model was represented by Chester Diocesan College where Arthur Riggs was the first principal. It was founded by John Sumner, later to be Archbishop of Canterbury, Edward Stanley, a Tory MP, and William Gladstone, then a liberal MP and of course a future Prime Minister. The Chester course was characterized by its scientific and practical nature. Students were actively involved in building the college and all of them were taught a trade, such as cabinet-making or book-binding. Day students were recruited from industry and commerce. The middle-class school attached to the college became an outstanding school of science. The inspectorate at the time described the Chester trainees as robust, healthy men, four of whom would weigh as much as five students at Battersea and six at St Mark's!

Over time the Battersea model came to dominate teacher training and the approach it promoted was influential until recently, as is shown by William Taylor's characterization of much of the initial teacher training of the 1970s:

> The emphasis on pastoral care; a residential tradition; awareness of the social and moral responsibilities of teachers and a distinct anxiety about academism, fears about over-emphasising relevance and practicality, a scepticism about technological advance (Taylor, 1984).

In the 1990s, as Richard Aldrich (1990) points out, much of the debate of the 1860s has a familiar ring to it. There is strong pressure today to make teacher training a more simple, direct, quasi-apprenticeship system, and to disengage it from the perceived high-flown and disturbing ideas and ideologies that come via higher education. On the other hand, there is a desire to recruit teachers that are academically able. If they are that, however, it is argued that there is no requirement for specific teacher training of a professional nature. Furthermore, there is still the practical, scientific and technological emphasis in teacher training. That emphasis is strongly present in the development of NCVQs and is influential in much of the competence-based approach to ITT.

Just where these debates will settle over time is unclear. Many factors other than philosophical and ideological arguments are likely to influence events. Among those will be teacher supply and demand. If as is forecast, the country emerges from economic recession into health and wealth again, it is possible that teaching will face particular and general shortages of supply. On the other hand, the signs are that there will be an over-supply of graduates in the labour market for some time to come.

Faced with supply problems even the most ideologically-driven governments bend to expediency. But however matters of supply and demand work out, we should not lose sight of the fact that the general drift and direction of government involvement in ITT over the past two decades has been away from the specifics of teaching quality and competence, even though they still feature in the rhetoric, and towards a much older, fundamental and difficult debate about who should teach; about the kind of people we think teachers ought to be; and what culture and values we believe they should be transmitting to the next generation.

These are important questions that every society needs to consider from time to time. They raise issues such as, 'What kind of people do parents, employers, pupils, governments and society at large want their teachers to be?'; 'What do they think they want them to do?', and above all, 'What kinds of training and links with higher education are needed to ensure that the status and standing of teaching and of the teaching profession are as high as they can be?'. Those are fundamental matters. The standing of teaching needs to be high to attract into teaching some of the best and brightest of each generation; to keep confident, competent and first-class practitioners in teaching; and to enable society to trust its teachers to make a stimulating and effective job of educating our children. If we fail to do these things, raising the standards of our education service and of pupil and student achievement will be a forlorn effort.

References

Aldrich, R (1990) 'The evolution of teacher education', in Graves, N (ed) *Initial Teacher Education*, London: Kogan Page.

Kay-Shuttleworth, J P (1862) *Four Periods of Public Education*, London: Longman.

Taylor, W (1984) 'The national context 1972–82', in Alexander, R, Craft, M and Lynch, J (eds) *Change in Teacher Education: Context and Provision Since Robbins*, London: Holt, Rinehart and Winston.

Chapter 2

Professionalism, Expertise and Control in Teacher Training

Rob Moore

Introduction

Both the definition of the teacher's role and the status of the teaching profession depend to a significant degree upon institutional relationships between the professional community and other groups and agencies involved in education. This chapter will examine the ways in which teachers as a professional community are located within such networks of relationships with other institutions and groups, and how those relationships construct the profession in different forms. Reform of teacher training and of education in general can be seen in terms of changes in these interrelationships and their justifications. Especially important in this respect are those groups which can be termed 'the gate-keepers' – groups or institutions which, by virtue of their regulative function, have the key role in defining what it is to *be* a teacher. These arrangements structure teachers' work and the distribution of responsibility and decision making between different groups. The Schools Curriculum and Assessment Authority (SCAA) and the proposed Teacher Training Agency (TTA) are major examples of 'gatekeepers'.

The question addressed in this chapter is how we can understand the proposed changes in teacher training in terms of these broader sets of relationships within which the teaching profession is located and which structure its form and status. The general trend since 1979 has been one which shifts the centre of gravity away from gatekeepers located within the educational system to ones located outside it. Hence the shift towards school-based training and the relative demotion of higher education has to be located within a broader framework which takes account of this central shift of power away from professional educators towards the central state and the market.

Paradigms and professionalism

Essentially, these relationships provide the teaching profession with principles for grounding its authority and its professional identity. Two major forms or 'paradigms' of teacher authority and professionalism based *within* education have dominated British education in the post-war period.

The first is that which defines 'the teacher' in terms of a relationship to knowledge. As the philosopher R S Peters put it, the teacher has authority by virtue of being an authority (ie in a subject). It is not simply the content of knowledge that is important but the rational principles and procedures whereby it is socially produced and assessed. In this instance, it is the academic community (or more precisely the rational, knowledge-creating principles and procedures which underpin it) which constitutes the gatekeeper. This paradigm is conventionally associated with educational 'traditionalism' and has been criticized as being overly 'academic' and élitist. However, there is no reason why a knowledge-based model should necessarily adopt this particular social form. I would argue that critics have been too preoccupied with the social implications of the 'traditional' model at the expense of the epistemological arguments of liberal philosophers such as Peters, Hirst and Bailey. I will use a version of this paradigm later in this chapter when discussing the relationship of teacher training to higher education.

The second form can be termed the 'educationalist' paradigm. Here, the teacher's authority is grounded in claims to expertise regarding 'the child' and the learning process. Its roots are in the Romantic tradition with its stress upon 'creativity' and 'discovery'. In the twentieth century it was underpinned by developmental child psychology. This 'child-centred' model is associated with 'progressivism' and has been the focus of considerable criticism. The changes in teacher training are frequently justified as eliminating the influence of this particular set of educationalist gatekeepers.

Conventionally, these paradigms are seen as radically opposed. The battle between traditionalism and progressivism has been an enduring feature of educational debates. However, there are a number of reasons why this view should be challenged. First, subject expertise and expertise in the educational process should be seen as equally necessary, complementary dimensions of the teacher's role. Secondly, traditionalism and progressivism share certain fundamental values in common. Both are liberal-humanist in the sense of seeing education as an intrinsic good, rather than simply a means to an end, and in being concerned with developing general states of moral consciousness such as rational autonomy, self-realization or character. Thirdly, they each provide grounds for professional autonomy, and claims to special expertise and the right to exercise judgement independent of political control.

It is a mistake to see the current reform of teacher training as a return to traditionalism at the expense of progressivism. In fact, these reforms reflect a challenge to the basic principles of liberal education *per se*, both progressive and traditional. The significant difference between these gatekeeping paradigms and the newly emerging one is that the new gatekeepers will no longer be within education, but will represent outside interests. It is the principle of professional autonomy which is at stake. Recent educational reform has been aimed at constructing an instrumental education directed towards the external ends of economic efficiency (the 'modernizers' competence-based skills model) and traditional values (neo-conservative 'back to basics'). The really significant division today is no longer between traditionalism and progressivism but between liberal education and its opponents.

School-based training and professional control

If it is established, the major gatekeeper within the newly emerging framework will be the TTA. It is designed to have the power to determine what is an acceptable course leading to qualified teacher status (QTS), and hence, what it is to be a teacher. It will be able to regulate school/HE partnerships. It may also play a powerful role in directing educational research funding and, thereby, control the research community. The proposed TTA will bring together under its control a range of functions previously dispersed across a number of different institutions, thereby centralizing control over training, research funding, and accreditation and evaluation. The term 'training agency' can be seen as indicative of a significant ideological shift which favours the rhetoric of vocational skills training rather than that of liberal education. The prospect of a narrowly vocationalized skills training for teachers must be seen as very real (FEU, 1982). The behavioural, prescriptive character of the competence approach makes it an ideal mechanism for control (Jones and Moore, 1993).

Superficially, school-centred courses could be interpreted as increasing the degree of *professional* control over teacher training. Education Minister Emily Blatch (1993), on announcing the second round of bidding for school-centred training courses, said that:

> Under the school-centred teacher training scheme, schools will have *real power* to decide how new members of the teaching profession should be trained.

However, if the TTA comes into being, the professional community will not itself be able to determine the form that training takes within the schools nor have the power or means to accredit it. School-based training will be subject to external regulation by the TTA. It is in controlling recruitment and regulating the professional body that professionalization within teaching has traditionally been weakest and where it departs most significantly from the models provided by medicine and law. The institutional arrangements for the profession to control training in any real sense do not exist and school-based training and the TTA do not bring them into being. More accurately, schools will simply be administering the TTA's model within the broader context of constraints constructed by government education policy.

The proposed shift to school-based training and the diminishing of the HE contribution can be located within a general ideological drive towards deprofessionalization and a challenge to professional status and autonomy as we have traditionally understood them. Particularly since the 1988 Education Reform Act and the establishing of the National Curriculum, teachers have demonstrated a growing awareness of this situation. The successful campaign against testing and the opposition expressed to the 'Mums Army' proposal are indicative of teachers' concern about the undermining of their professional expertise, judgement and autonomy. Hence the questions arise:

- How much power will the profession have, in reality, to decide how new members should be trained?
- Towards what model of 'the teacher' will that training be directed?
- How does the relationship with HE affect the model of professionalism?

The New Right and Professionalism

The New Right's opposition towards the traditional, liberal model of the profession takes three main forms.

First, *the market argument* sees the professional group as representing 'producer capture' acting against the interest of consumers, and professional ideals and values as little more than rhetoric disguising monopolistic self-interest. The existence of professional groups and their capacity to control the supply of services distorts the free play of market forces. A major aspect of government policy since 1979 has been to break down professional and other forms of 'closure' and introduce the 'discipline of the market', especially into the public sector.

Second, *the 'values' argument* focuses upon two aspects of professional culture. There is its liberal, anti-commercial ethic associated with the values of service and disinterestedness. In education, opposition to such values is related to the move away from a comprehensive, integrated public service towards a differentiated, competitive, one. At a more general political level it is associated with a shift from treating individuals as citizens with (universal) rights to treating them as consumers with (economically varying) demands in relation to services.

There is also a more specific antipathy towards the *expertise* exercised by professional groups. The dismissal of expert opinion has been a feature of New Right political rhetoric. The views of professional educators especially have been subject to this treatment and the exclusion of professional opinion was a notable feature of the National Curriculum working parties. An attempt has been made to replace the liberal professional ethic and its claims to authority with an 'enterprise culture' and entrepreneurial values.

Third, *the political argument* is less explicitly stated but of considerable significance. Traditionally, professional communities have been seen as making a special contribution to the maintenance of liberal democracy. They were seen as an important part of the countervailing forces of a pluralistic democracy, balancing the power of the central state. In the immediate post-war period, this arrangement was deliberately nurtured as a bulwark against totalitarianism. Strong, autonomous professional communities were seen as a crucial ingredient of the political culture and respected, independent contributors to policy formation and public debate.

Since 1979, government policies have attempted to disestablish professional cultures and institutions across the range of social and economic life – from finance and law, through the welfare state, local government and the civil service to the police force. Alongside the constraints on trade union activity, this represents a general policy of legal and institutional change which weakens the power of occupational groups. Especially in the public sector, changes in the institutional arrangements of control have led to the decline of professional autonomy, an increase in the powers of central state and the introduction of quasi-market mechanisms. The restructuring of teacher training is associated with a diminution of the professional status of teachers and an impoverishment of their role. Against the background of such hostility towards professional groups and liberal values, it would be mistaken to interpret these changes as having anything to do with enhancing teacher professionalism.

Professionalism and partnership

The shift to school-based training and the changing relationship to HE disconnects teachers from the bodies of academic knowledge and research which can provide the basis for authoritative, professional autonomy and expertise and the claim to a legitimate role in policy formation. The craft skills of teaching (or any other occupation) are always most effectively acquired on-the-job as they crucially involve the acquisition of the tacit skills of the occupational culture. There is nothing at all wrong with the view that teacher training should involve a major school-based component and that the schools themselves may be the best institutions to organize it. It is using school-based training as a *substitute* for initial professional training that is disputed.

The purpose of the HE aspect of teacher training should be to provide in an academically demanding, rigorous and systematic fashion the bodies of theoretical knowledge and cumulative research findings of value and interest to teachers on the basis of which they can claim expertise in the field of education in addition to being effective practitioners in the classroom. It is a mistake for HE teacher trainers to ground their claims to authority in an appeal to practice – by the logic of that argument it will always be the case that the schools could possibly do it better. The genuinely distinctive contribution of HE to the training of teachers and their further professional development is in providing access to the bodies of academic knowledge, scholarship and research of relevance to them in their professional practice. It is on this basis that we can see a proper complementarity between HE and the teaching profession.

This should not, however, be seen in terms of a relationship of theory to practice (see below). Scholarship and research are as much forms of practice as classroom teaching and all teaching involves theoretical assumptions. We should be seeking a productive working relationship between two independent bodies of practitioners and their distinctive forms of expertise. The major function of HE in initial teacher training (ITT) is to provide teachers with a window into academic scholarship and research, and to foster the appreciation that to be a teacher in a full professional sense is to be an informed expert in the field of education as well as an effective practitioner in a classroom.

Theory and Rhetoric

The move to school-based training is explicitly justified in terms of an attack on theory. The Secretary of State for Education, John Patten, said in a lecture delivered to the Conservative Political Centre in October 1993 that:

> ...we are ensuring that teacher training is precisely that, training – undertaken as much as possible in the school – and not wasted studying dated and irrelevant texts on theory. To that end, we have recently announced the first wholly school-based teacher training scheme.

Given that no one would seriously suggest that students should devote themselves to the study of 'dated and irrelevant texts', Patten here appears to be dismissing theory *per se*, however up-to-date or relevant. He is also clear as to what a preparation for teaching is to be – *training*, 'precisely that'. If we review the many tirades against 'theories' in teacher training (eg in the reading debate), more often than not they turn out to be disputes over the relative advantages and disadvantages of particular teaching methods. *Theory* is usually noticeable by its absence. On the one hand, the theoretical underpinnings of teaching methods (both those attacked and those advocated) are rarely made explicit or rigorously examined and on the other, the theories which link certain social conditions – for example 'the decline in respect for authority', 'lack of economic competitiveness' – with a particular style of teaching, remain deeply buried and unacknowledged.

Patten provides an example of this. The reconstruction of teacher training is part of the '...task of stopping the rot in education which had set in in the 1960s' (ibid). Buried within this comment is an hypothesis open, in principle, to examination. The Secretary of State appears to be harbouring a theory – a systematic set of ideas about what was and is empirically the case and about the underlying causal links between certain sets of events or conditions. We can assume that the 'rot' has something to do with progressivism for he tells us that 'Too many people have left our teacher training colleges...conversant in the ways of "progressive" orthodoxy but without knowing how to teach children to read' (ibid). What does this actually *mean*; where is the *evidence*?

As critical references in the press to Plowden indicate, educational reforms are represented in both the popular imagination and for politicians and policy-makers as the replacement of progressivism by a more traditional model. Within this discourse, progressivism is associated with the group referred to as the 'liberal educational establishment' or the 'trendy experts' –

the educationalist gatekeepers based in teacher training, the local education authorities and HM Inspectorate. Given the power of this progressive *versus* traditional dichotomy and the way in which it shapes the national discourse of education, it is important to stress its limitations as a way of describing what actually goes on in classrooms. Major research programmes in the early 1970s such as those of Bennett and Galton found that the labels traditional and progressive were of little value in describing what teachers actually *did* in class, regardless of their own willingness to adopt the labels. Indeed, 'teaching style' as such is not now seen as being of major significance compared with other factors such as school organization (Gipps, 1992).

Whatever problems there might be in schools and society, the idea that they are caused by 'progressivism' is difficult to credit — typically researchers have great difficulty in finding enough 'progressivism' to constitute a reasonable sample for study let alone serve as the basis for a general theory of social and economic decline! This does not imply that the real problem is not *enough* progressivism, but that the phenomenon itself is more a figment of political rhetoric than a substantive feature of educational reality. This well illustrates the problems that arise when politically expedient 'theories' are protected from examination by academic scholarship and research.

In terms of educational research, we can say that the movement, over the past twenty years, from 'teaching style' to 'school effects' should have led to a general questioning of the status of the terms 'traditional' and 'progressive'. However, the terms have a broader, symbolic role in marking out positions linked with other discourses in society. In this fashion, educational debates are associated with wider areas of social concern. It is clear, for instance, that within the public domain traditionalism *versus* progressivism has as much to do with views about moral order, discipline and authority in *society* as with what actually goes on in schools. In this way, the co-opting of educational issues by broader ideological agendas, distorts and confuses educational debate.

Theory and 'common sense'

The idea that some people (eg progressive teacher trainers) have theories and others (eg Secretaries of State for Education) do not is untenable. The lecture by Patten quoted above contains a number of theories developed to varying degrees of explicitness. Indeed, it contains one concerning the social causes and effects of functional illiteracy, which is developed in some detail.

Patten reveals himself to be no mean theorist when he chooses! But this is precisely the point. What is going on here is a picking and choosing between theories according to political and administrative expediency. Theory is explicitly denied but its authority implicitly invoked to advance a particular cause.

What the attack on theory illustrates is the arbitrary and opportunistic way in which theory is incorporated into public debates and political rhetoric. This device operates by opposing theory with the alternative of common sense. The latter is implicitly taken as what any sensible person knows to be really the case. Theory by contrast, is presented as self-indulgent, out-of-touch, unworldly and narcissistic. Beneath the surface of such arguments is a set of claims, both empirical and causal, which are open to rigorous formulation and testing. It is *in fact* the case that particular things have occurred and is it plausible that they have *caused* the effects being attributed to them and *how*? In other words, the argument against theory is *itself* a theory – if we do this rather than that, this will follow. It makes claims about what is empirically the case and about causal relationships and hypothesizes about the effects of change.

The appeal to practice and common sense – to the practitioner against the theoretician – is fundamentally untenable for two reasons. First, it pretends that it is not itself a theory at all and, second, it attempts to protect itself from the kind of rigorous, critical questioning to which all theories have to be subjected. The use of the terms 'common sense' and 'practice' is simply a means of protecting a politically preferred theory. It is important to be clear about what is happening here. Presenting teaching as common sense privileges and imposes one particular model of professional expertise as the only acceptable one. The key question is: acceptable to whom? Essentially, the underlying issue is one of control. Which groups acquire the power to control expertise and its forms and, especially, its capacity for reflexive criticism?

In summary, we can say this of the attack on theory. First, the term as such is used in an imprecise and inaccurate way, and is usually applied to methods rather than theories. Second, the assertions of the anti-theorists are themselves theories. By calling their own theories 'common sense' the anti-theorists attempt to exempt them from critical appraisal. We are all theorists whether or not we recognize it. Third, the distinction between theory and common sense does not stand up for not only is common sense ideologically constructed but it is also inevitably theory laden. The opposition to theory is selective and opportunistic, and in fact has to do with promoting one set of politically favoured theories over others and one group of theorists over the rest. Essentially this debate is to do with political manoeuvring to secure the dominance of a new set of gatekeepers who, in contrast to the academics and professional educationalists, actively seek to exclude their own theories from critical scrutiny and open debate, and so indicate a reluctance to accept outside interference in the policy-making process. By attempting to disconnect teachers from the academic community it sets out to secure a monopoly of educational theory for the political policy-makers. The great danger is that the body of academic work, rather than being open to the profession, will be selectively filtered by the politicians and policy-makers according to their own particular interests, as Patten's lecture indicates.

Professionalism and Expertise

I have suggested that the relationship between the HE and the professional contributions to ITT should not be confused with a distinction between theory and practice. I want to indicate some further points about the relationship between the two by developing an alternative distinction between the expertise of production and the expertise of application. I will use this distinction as the basis for discussing the relationship between training, teacher professionalism and knowledge.

The debate around teacher professionalism is complicated. First, the definition of 'profession' as such is problematic (Perkin, 1989), and second, teaching obviously departs in significant ways from the traditional institutional models provided by medicine and law. I do not intend to review these problems in detail; suffice it to say that whatever the definitional problems, teachers certainly think of themselves as professionals and have a strong collective sense of what this should entail in terms of individual and group status.

Central to this is the idea of autonomy both at the individual level of classroom work and more broadly in terms of respect for the profession's views in matters of educational policy. In both these senses, professionalism relates to the exercising of informed judgement. At the individual level, the teacher should be allowed to exercise judgement in his or her own classroom and, at the collective level, the practitioner community should be accorded a special status in the consideration of educational concerns.

Implicit within this is an assumption that the profession possesses a body of knowledge relating to its practice on the basis of which its views deserve special consideration and without which one cannot properly be said to *be* a teacher. I will refer to this special relationship between knowledge and practice as 'expertise' and I am going to argue that it is this expertise which is crucially at stake in the restructuring of the relationships of teacher training.

Knowledge, practice and expertise

Expertise, in the sense that I want to use the term, can be taken as referring to a systematically refined set of practices exercised by a recognized community of practitioners for a specially designated social purpose. Understood in this way, expertise entails a distinction between it and everyday practices which might be seen as directed towards a similar end, and also between the group which possesses the expertise and the lay community. An illustration of this is the relationship between DIY in the home (however enthusiastically pursued) and the same type of work carried out by a professional builder, decorator, carpenter or whatever.

In most cases, expertise is a specialized, developed form of things that most of us could do at some time or other in our lives, although the availability of the services of experts can relieve us of the necessity of actually doing so. Few of us would opt for DIY disposal of deceased relatives rather than turn to the services of an undertaker! The skills of dealing with the experts take over from personal attempts to exercise the skills themselves.

Expertise is legitimated by a number of principles at differing levels of abstraction and generality. First of all, experts can claim a superior level of practice simply because they have more practice – they do it more often. Second, they also have training – they acquire the body of skill in a systematic fashion. Third, there is social recognition of the right to claim expertise – a 'license' or mandate to practice. In combination, these features produce a crucial, distinctive feature of expertise: its detachment from particular local, everyday settings and its specialization. For instance, occasionally I practice certain of the skills associated with the building trades, but the skills I use in, say, attempting to erect bookshelves, are only an *ad hoc* and limited selection of the total set of associated skills possessed by an expert. Furthermore, when I perform this task I do so in the role of householder, father, friend or husband. I do not *become* a specialized book-shelf erector let alone a carpenter! I perform the task as an adjunct of some other facet of my social role or self-image.

The lay practice is heavily contextualized and situated within a particular pragmatic context. By contrast, the expert possesses a wider, systematic body of skills and the experience to apply them selectively and effectively to any particular situation. Although I might become adept at nurturing the particular plants I grow in my own back garden, in contrast to the horticultural expert, I can claim no authority as far as different plants in other people's back gardens are concerned. This relative detachment or decontextualization of expertise provides the basis for its systematic development. The community of experts can turn its attention to the rationalization, refinement and further development of its body of knowledge and skill. This possibility profoundly affects the character of the professional community and the relationship of expertise to commonsense or everyday knowledge.

There are two particularly important features of this. The first is that of reflexivity; that is, the process of critical, systematic reflection upon the practices themselves, essentially asking the question, 'How do they work?' Reflexivity provides the basis for theory and the development of a deeper understanding of underlying principles and causal processes. It becomes associated with the development of powerful sets of procedures which generate understandings of basic processes and the capacity to develop new ways of doing things. Second, there is, historically, a tendency for an additional level of specialization to occur between those who practice this critically reflexive examination of expertise and those who practice its application. We can recognize this process in terms of the formation of powerful foundation disciplines mainly located within the university in modern society, and a proliferation of bodies of knowledge and procedures come into being which increasingly have their own distinctive institutional settings, interests and developmental dynamics (following the logic of the discipline).

I will refer to these forms of expertise as 'disciplines' of *knowledge production* as distinct from professional expertise concerned with *applications*. This is not equivalent to a distinction between theory and practice. Professional expertise is intrinsically theoretical and, equally, the disciplines are themselves forms of practice. Rather, the distinction has to do with the primary concerns of the two forms of expertise: production and application. The relationship between these two, interdependent, forms of expertise and their practitioners is the key issue under consideration.

Critical Reflection – The Third Practice

The distinction between production and application should not be seen as implying an élitist separation between those who produce new knowledge and those who 'merely' apply it. The expertise of application entails its own genuinely creative, reflexive activity. Whereas the expertise of production lies very much in working within a particular theoretical or research paradigm (following the logic of the discipline), that of application has more to do with the creative synthesizing of such work.

Reality is always more complex than theory. Theory illuminates reality in particular, partial ways, but never exhausts it. The application of theory should, ideally, reveal the limitations of both established practices and of theories themselves. New theories throw the implicit assumptions of established practices into sharp relief − revealing their taken-for-granted principles and underlying theoretical status. At the same time, the pragmatic eclecticism of application highlights both the partiality of any particular theory and the possibility of synthesizing ideas and perspectives across the boundaries of disciplines and paradigms in new and original ways. We could say that the creative dialogue between production and application is that in which each reveals the blind-spots of the other.

The mutually supportive relationship between teachers and researchers is one in which they engage together in the common activity of critical reflection on their respective practices utilizing the resources of theory and application in the shared interest of deepening their respective knowledge and effectiveness. We can think of this as a 'third practice', or form of expertise, which those of production and application can share in common and which is the precondition for the healthy development of both. Ideally teacher training should provide the foundation for this third practice, establishing the venues, habits and conventions of its common culture and a level playing field between its participants in terms of knowledge and skill.

Research into classroom teaching reveals that teachers do not (contrary to the simplistic view of the traditional *versus* progressive dichotomy) dogmatically apply a single teaching method; they draw eclectically upon a repertoire of styles and skills. The expertise of the professional teacher lies precisely in the ability to construct an ensemble of methods and approaches as need arises. Practitioners should be able to draw selectively upon the disciplines, taking from them those things that they judge to be relevant and adapting and reassembling them as appears appropriate. It is not the business of sociologists, psychologists, philosophers etc., to tell teachers how to teach. Rather, in following their own (intra-disciplinary) interests in education, they should ensure that their research and scholarship is available to teachers and that the institutional spaces and opportunities exist for productive dialogue between the two communities based upon the common enterprise of critical reflection.

Conclusion

The attack on theory and the attempt to separate the expertise of production from that of application on the basis of a spurious distinction between theory and practice, is in reality an ideologically motivated attempt to privilege, protect and impose one particular theory − that embedded within the model of practice being legitimated as common sense.

The key relationship is that between two distinctive but complementary forms of expertise − those of production and application. As I have stressed, this is not equivalent to a distinction between theory and practice. Both are forms of practice and all practice is underpinned by theory. It is in this that we see the most serious consequence of attempting to separate the expertise of application from that of production. What is most significant and distinctive about expertise in the way that I am describing it is not its content but its reflexivity; its capacity for critical reflection. It is not just that the practitioner community could lose access to a body of knowledge produced by the academic community but, more significantly, access to the principles and procedures through which that knowledge is produced.

What is (or should be) shared between these two communities of practitioners, and is the precondition for dialogue and the ultimate ground of their respective expertise, is precisely the complex set of critical, analytic and synthesizing skills which make up reflexivity − the practice of theory. This, I suggest, should be seen as constituting the third practice which is shared in common and the cultivation of which, as a general attitude of mind and an approach to life, is what education in the liberal tradition is ultimately all about.

Acknowledgement

I would like to thank John Beck, Sheila Miles and Jenny Daniels for their constructive comments on draft versions of this chapter.

References

Blatch, E (1993) *Department for Education News*, 29 September.
Further Education Unit (1982) *Competency in Teaching*, London: FEU.
Gipps, C (1992) *Effective Primary Teaching*, London: Tufnell.
Jones, L and Moore, R (1993) 'Education, competence and the control of expertise', *British Journal of Sociology of Education*, 14, 4.
Perkin, H (1989) *The Rise of Professional Society*, London: Routledge.

Chapter 3

The Language of Partnership

Terry Allsop

You say you want me to supervise a student teacher coming for block
teaching practice next term. That's pretty good news: I'll have lots of extra
free lessons. But the down side is that I'll have to pick up the pieces after he's
gone.

Far fetched and anachronistic, you may say, but all the parts of this com-
posite 'quotation' can still be heard regularly in schools today. Despite the
designation of schools and training institutions as 'partners' in training, it is
still possible to find the attitudes which were noted in 1988 in a study of the
experiences of student teachers, that practising teachers value them because:

> ...of the relief from virtual non-stop classroom teaching which a student
> teacher may provide, and the welcome opportunity to catch up with
> ....preparation of lessons and the marking of pupils' work. (Leighton and
> Aldrich, 1988).

The purpose of this chapter is to explore the language of partnership as new
patterns of school–higher education collaboration are created. Is there old,
redundant language? Is a new, more appropriate language emerging? Or,
more generally, what does the language register used in relation to training
to teach between schools and higher education institutions suggest about the
nature of the partnership between them? Fairly arbitrarily, with some over-
lapping, the analysis is presented in five sections, as follows, with concluding
comments:

- the procedural language of partnership
- the language of the professional players
- the response of the school staff
- the experience of the beginning teachers
- the language of assessment.

An immediate point of interest is the designation of the beginning teacher.
Terms like 'student' and 'student teacher' cause difficulties because school

pupils are now frequently termed 'students'. They also indicate the status of the student in the school. In school-based training the beginning teacher is an associate member of the school staff and this is acknowledged in some institutions such as Keele University where students are known as 'associate teachers'. But such terms are inappropriate if the beginner's attachment to the school is of a duration of just a few weeks on 'block practice' when they can only be seen as birds of passage. But it is not clear that terms like 'associate teacher' or 'intern' (the Oxford Internship Scheme designation with which the writer works reasonably comfortably on a day-to-day basis and which experience provides the practical grounding for this chapter) deal sufficiently with issues to do with the status of a professional learner within a partnership involving two institutions with professional staff.

The Procedural Language of Partnership

Circular 24/89 from the then DES makes the first strong official pronouncement about the benefits of partnership, after a decade during which only the more adventurous explored that possibility. It said definitively and without discussion that:

> Close cooperation between schools, local education authorities and initial teacher training institutions leads to better training of student teachers for their future careers and provides valuable staff development for institutions and schools. Where possible, institutions should build long-term partnerships with individual schools which will foster collaboration and training opportunities.

In the light of more recent formulations, the language of what follows in the 1989 Circular appears well balanced, even enlightened, focusing as it does on the mutual benefits for staff of HE institutions and schools, as well as for the beginning teacher:

> Serving teachers stand to gain through contacts with developments in curriculum thinking and from the fresh insights of the students and teacher trainers with whom they work.
> Tutors, as well as practising teachers, are seen as role models by students. If tutors maintain and develop their teaching experience they will ensure that the training which they provide for students reflects the changing curricula and needs of schools.

The effect of Circular 24/89 was that the language used in descriptors of some PGCE courses began to change significantly. A sample 1989 course handbook talks of ' ...our policy of bringing the schools into a closer partnership', though even this could be read as having paternalistic overtones. But the same handbook also talks of ' ...the heavy *demands* made on schools for teaching practice places' (my emphasis), a confusion which reflects the transitions taking place. However, even as late as 1993, scrutiny of some PGCE course brochures reveals no mention of partnership or of roles for teachers in the training process.

Having officially endorsed partnership in 1989, the government redefined it in an acutely destabilizing sequence of pronouncements during 1992. These started with the Secretary of State's speech of 4 January, which was made policy by the publication of Circular 9/92 by the DfE, and by a further note of guidance published in November by CATE, all of which use a sharper tone in presenting a very different perspective on the notion of partnership. The Secretary of State picked up from the HMI report (1991) on school-based training 'the need for strong and clearly understood links between HE tutors, their students and the teachers who are helping to train them' and deliberately shifted the balance in potential partnerships by indicating that:

> ... the whole process of teacher training needs to be based on a more equal partnership between school teachers and tutors in institutions, *with the schools playing a much bigger part* (my emphasis).

Readers will be able to draw continua of partnership relating to their own institutions, be they schools or HE institutions and make their own judgements as to where their own experience places them. The rhetoric of Circular 9/92 provides a strong and immediate definition of the nature of the partnerships envisaged, a definition which suggests that there is very little scope for the kind of discourse and dialogue which might reasonably be thought to be essential to the balance of responsibilities within an equal partnership. Against the background of the historical imbalance in relationships in teacher training between HE institutions and schools (LEAs have totally dropped out of the picture), this is hardly surprising, but the most important consequence has been that partnership negotiations have been dominated by the vexed question of resource distribution rather than focusing on the nature of the contributions to be made by the partners. Conceptualizing a partnership in school-based or school-focused training is not a straightforward task, nor is operationalizing it achieved in weeks or even months, as we shall see from the Oxford experience.

Already, in scrutinizing the planning of PGCE courses for 1993/4, it is possible to see the shift which has been politically induced by the government, in the ways in which communication between HE institutions and schools proceeds, in relation both to course advertising and course planning. This has been promoted by the requirement that 'partnership agreements' shall be prepared for each course. In the case of one HE institution which had made important planning steps in relation to partnership with full involvement of local schools, headteachers and LEAs *prior* to the 9/92 requirements, such that, '...we have already developed a course which requires clear and complementary contributions from both the schools and the university...', the outline role descriptions for the partners are given as:

Walford University/School Partnership –
A Model for Secondary PGCE Teacher Education

that the university will provide a full programme of method work and complementary studies for students, and will support students' work in school through regular visits from method and seminar tutors... The university will provide and fund a programme of preparation for teachers to enable them to fulfil their roles;

that the school will, during school-based weeks, provide students with access to classes and will arrange for supervising teachers (subject mentors) to spend one lesson per week with their pair of students, and for the professional tutors to spend one morning a week with the whole group of students.

While this description of roles in a developing partnership follows the general trend through the 1980s towards greater engagement of school teachers in the in-school preparation of beginning teachers and retains a significant role for university tutors in schools, it does not match the language of the CATE amplification of Circular 9/92, which tilts responsibility for the school experience of the beginning teacher almost completely away from the university tutor, except marginally in relation to assessment. In effect the CATE document writes out the role of 'subject tutor' or 'curriculum tutor'. In the pilot schemes of wholly school-centred initial teacher training (SCITT) currently being rushed through by the DfE, the documentation for those seeking to bid for inclusion in such schemes virtually eliminates higher education institutions from the training process, except by invitation 'if necessary'. Is this the language of partnership? Have 'partnership agreements', so recently introduced to the scene, already become outdated language?

The points made in this section can be summarized: the government has sought first to introduce partnership into all HEI-school links (of which some few cases already existed) and then to impose a form of training which has moved beyond partnership to an imbalance in the responsibility for training in favour of the schools. The language of institutional prospectuses suggests that there has been a move towards partnership in rhetoric at least, but it is too early to note institutional reactions to more recent government requirements for a school-dominated form of training.

The Language of the Professional Players

So where does all this leave, on the one hand, the burgeoning ranks of mentors and professional tutors who are school-based and, on the other, the threatened species variously titled curriculum tutors, link tutors, general tutors, subject method tutors, associate tutors and education tutors who are HE-based? Well, put simply, the former are flourishing and multiplying (and this is not the place to explore the emerging interpretations of mentoring), while the latter are scrambling around trying to make sense of a world where they are apparently unloved, without a role, and even more important, without resources. But the world has not gone entirely crazy, and there is emerging a genuine practice of partnership, where the functions of schools and HE-based professionals are being clearly delineated. In the best practice, the beginning teacher is clearly placed at the centre of a network of professionals, each of whom has distinct, complementary functions which are explicitly set out in language which all the partners understand as in the example just quoted, since they have all been involved in the development phase. In many institutions the description of these functions has outstripped both the understanding and the practice of them, and this is perhaps particularly acute in the case of mentors working with beginning teachers in their classrooms. After all, ten years ago, who had even thought of using the term 'mentor' in a teacher education context? That is a short time in which to achieve coincidence between the conceptual understandings, institutional arrangements and forms of action which are contained within the term 'mentor'.

A brief excursion through the Oxford experience may be helpful here because it shows how long it takes to achieve a common language which reflects a shared outlook. For six years now, each pair of interns has related to four professionals, as shown in Figure 3.1. The crucial communications have always been perceived to be between the subject specialists (mentor and curriculum tutor) and those with whole-school responsibilities (general tutor and professional tutor).

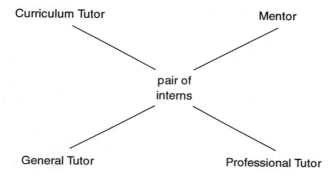

CURRICULUM WORK
The professional development of interns in relation to classroom practice

Curriculum Tutor   Mentor

pair of
interns

General Tutor   Professional Tutor

Professional development of interns in relation to whole-school issues
PROFESSIONAL DEVELOPMENT PROGRAMME

Figure 3.1 *Responsibilities in the Oxford Internship Scheme*

As was suggested above, the mentor role involves taking on the detailed, day-to-day support of the intern in his or her subject classroom. Induction into this role has been shared increasingly equally by experienced curriculum tutors and experienced mentors, and these common experiences, together with the agendas of regular meetings in subject groupings between mentors and curriculum tutors have generated a common shared language of support for interns, over a period of six years of interactions in school and university settings. Nevertheless and although curriculum tutors are generally highly visible in internship schools, a mentor can still recently write of the curriculum tutor as 'our external partner', thus implying the serious part of the partnership was with the school.

The general tutor/professional tutor partnership is at first sight perhaps less intensive, as it takes the form of responsibility for the whole-school professional development programme for about ten interns, delivered in both school and university. The professional interactions are most fully tested in the school-based part of the programme, where the emphasis is properly put on the school's policies and approaches to a range of issues. The general tutor has the consistently sensitive task of making comparative inputs to the discourse of training within the school, while not belittling the school's own practice. The professional tutor has a major role in mediation between interns, mentors, other teachers, headteacher, parents, etc. She or he is well placed to measure the quality of the absorption and acceptance of the beginning teachers into the whole-school environment, and to act to promote this when and where necessary.

At least two quite new groupings of interested professionals are emerging in the internship scheme. Within schools, the meeting of subject mentors, convened by the professional tutor, is increasingly seen as one of the standing committees of the school, which creates its own discourse about initial teacher education within the school. This is then transmitted through subject departments. The termly meeting, in the higher education institution, of all the professional tutors of internship schools has developed its own dynamic and concerns. Typically, professional tutors are senior members of staff, although by no means all belong to senior management teams; some have ready access to the corridors of power, others do not. In virtually all cases they have deliberately chosen to make a significant professional investment in an area of work which would not traditionally be seen to be of high status in the hierarchy or life of the school. One of the consequences for the HE institution is the emergence of a coherent voice *across* schools within the partnership, which sometimes tests the interpretation of partnership in relation to decision making. A simple example would be the reluctance of professional tutors, as speakers for the schools, to accept the notion that beginning teachers need to spend time sharing experiences outside school even after their period of full-time work in schools has been under way for some time. This is usually phrased in the form of 'It's too disruptive for their timetables', and is echoed by many of the beginning teachers!

This section has noted the way in which, through working together, schools and the university department have developed a common language with which they feel comfortable and which acts to define their relationships and the tasks that each can expect of the other. But the development of such a language only occurs over time.

The Response of the School Staff

Student teachers should sit at the edge of the staff room along with other non-permanent members of staff (Member of school staff to beginning teacher, 1993).

In general, consultation and advice from staff not connected with mentoring was excellent (Oxford intern, 1993).

Teachers in any one school are likely to have three levels of involvement in work with beginning teachers: significant responsibility as mentors, some work in their own classrooms with beginning teachers, no formally structured interactions at all. The responses of the third group − of which two contrasting examples are given above − are of particular interest, as they give some indication of the extent to which partnership in initial teacher education has become embedded in the culture of the whole school − an estimable target.

At best, the whole staff will be formally introduced to the structures and practices which will make the partnership a reality, and which will make clear that the beginning teachers do themselves have a significant, although time-limited, commitment to the school. This will mean that the headteacher greets the beginning teachers by making clear to them that they are 'a part of the staff' and that the Staff Guide indicates that 'Interns are accepted as an integral part of the school'. But the reactions of the members of staff who do not work directly with the beginning teachers are not always positive. The hoary chestnuts of space in the staff room, the missing coffee mugs, the provision of pigeon holes for the beginning teachers, excessive use of photocopying facilities ('They make far too many worksheets in their first flush of enthusiasm') all provide fertile ground for expressed or smouldering irritation. Much more important is the public situation where a pupil, speaking to a member of staff, refers to a beginning teacher not known by name to the member of staff, whose response of 'Oh! You mean the student teacher' is less than helpful. The following comments which were culled from a recent meeting of professional tutors give a flavour of the tension sometimes experienced in schools as a consequence of taking interns:

> This group's already been used four times (Class teacher to professional tutor).
> I find myself having to persuade parents that having students teaching their kids is a good thing (Professional tutor).
> Is it fair to have children doing assessed coursework being taught by an intern? (Parent to professional tutor).
> Interns get blamed for everything! (Professional tutor).
> It's *your* intern who is smoking! (Teacher to professional tutor).

A strange, but very prevalent view is that the beginning teacher should 'feel the pain' of teaching the full timetable of a teacher. This manifests itself in a number of ways, the most striking being the importance to the schools of continuity once the beginning teacher is present in school on a full-time basis. There is reluctance to concede a programme structure which allows the beginning teacher concurrent short periods of reflection outside the school environment, and there is reluctance to take back classes when the beginning teacher has other tasks to complete – 'When you are a full-time teacher ......!'.

These comments suggest that being a partnership school even in a well-established scheme can have its problems. Inevitably, interns or students will disrupt the smooth running of the school in some respects. In 1993/4, the visitations of Ofsted inspection teams to internship schools has created an interesting dilemma for some: should the interns continue to teach classes as normal during the week of an inspection? Some have said 'Yes, of course'. Others responded by taking interns off classes for that week. The reader may wish to speculate about the relative levels of confidence in the partnership.

The Experience of the Beginning Teachers

I thought I would be treated like a second-class citizen within the bastions of the staff room, where I just knew no one would ever know my name, least of all use it. And as for anyone ever considering that my input into the science department would ever be more than a total nuisance and a complete disruption, well, it just couldn't be! How wrong I was! My first impression of the school, aside from the size, the noise and the sheer volume of people who trod its corridors, was one of friendliness and understanding. We met our mentors in very congenial surroundings, alongside the tutors who were already becoming receptors of a large amount of dependence. We were reassured, supported, cared about, it seemed, and the last impression I received was that we could ever be a nuisance or a disruption. In fact, we were made to feel of use, as if our very presence was of benefit to the school, and not just because we were another pair of hands. We were even given our own pigeon-holes, and our own photocopying number ... it was this last gesture which convinced me, I am here and they want me to be! (Oxford Intern, 1993).

This section is based almost entirely on the views and perspectives of 15 Oxford interns, writing and talking about their experiences in June 1993, at the very end of their PGCE year. As the above lengthy quotation shows, these can be very positive indeed.

The interns all found it almost impossible to articulate what had been their expectations of their roles in school prior to arrival on the course. They had already spent nearly three weeks in school, chiefly in observing mode, and so there was some initial and very real surprise at the extent to which they had been integrated into the body of the staff in their internship school. Early messages they received were almost wholly positive. They were always referred to as interns, not as student teachers, and were never introduced to pupils as student teachers. In many cases, integration into the staff room was initially difficult, '...as much due to intern hesitancy as any staff attitude', and this was definitely not helped in one case by a professional tutor who indicated an area of the staffroom·as 'That is usually the interns' table' – a comment which inhibited interns from mixing with colleagues in subject departments as their confidence grew later on. And what should ten interns do in a school new to internship, when ten new chairs are purchased for the staff room and sited in an area separated from the rest of the room by the main channel of movement?

The following snippets of interns' comments give a flavour of the way in which they perceived their situation. They reflect their growing commitment to the school and a pride and excitement in 'becoming a teacher'. But they also express anxiety and vulnerability. Its difficult to be 'professional' all the time.

> We were involved throughout in staff INSET, in extracurricular activities, in parent consultations and in staff social activities.
> There was a feeling as the year progressed of being a 'teacher' in school and a 'student' in the university. Possibly the school had a greater trust in our professional qualities than the university.
> On the front cover of a pupil's exercise book: Teacher – Mr. Higgins, Intern – Ms Khan.
> In a parents' evening, working alongside the subject teacher, it was necessary to be assertive to gain the attention of the parent. However, most parents did value my comments.
> Sometimes there was a frosty atmosphere in certain staff rooms. This was generated by particular members of staff.
> Caroline (intern) eating chocolate biscuit outside the staff room received the comment from another teacher – 'Oh honestly, I've just told off some pupils for eating!'
> There was an acceptance by pupils that we were real teachers even though mentors were present in many lessons.

As for the pupils, they simply said what they have always have said about student teachers:

> We need to be taught properly. We're fed up with students!
> You're only a supply teacher!
> Do we have to have Mr — again? Why are you leaving?

The Language of Assessment

The traditional assumption has been that the responsibility for the assessment of the beginning teacher has lain primarily with the higher education institution, the outcome being an award of its degree or certificate. This has been directly coupled to the granting of Qualified Teacher Status, a licence to teach. The involvement of teachers in assessment has been very varied, and the status of their contribution to the outcome of the process distinctly unclear. There has probably been a good deal of acquiescence to the status quo on both sides, with schools, in part properly, seeing it as not being their business to get involved in marking assignments, but then grumbling quietly that higher education institutions are insufficiently tough in their judgements concerning effective classroom practice. It seems likely that the reverse may be the case, with school teachers being most reluctant to put forward a failing grade on school experience for a student with whom they have worked for several weeks or months! But as HMI (1991) have indicated, it is probably quite common to find that 'Senior teachers ...have been given little or no opportunity to participate fully in the assessment of students'. Scrutiny of the assessment frameworks published in course handbooks for secondary PGCE courses prior to 1992 reveals virtually no evidence of teacher involvement in the process; the beginning teacher is being assessed by higher education tutors for a qualification of a higher education institution.

How then are we to think about assessment in the context of a partnership in training? The CATE Note of Guidance issued in November 1992 gives us some assistance:

> Normally: Schools will have a leading responsibility for assessing student competences in subject application and classroom skills... Whilst higher education institutions will be responsible for ensuring that students are assessed for the award of qualifications.

But these statements simply set up another tough set of questions:

- While acknowledging that teachers working as mentors will have by far the greatest day-to-day knowledge of the beginning teacher's classroom skills, how will they:
  - develop skills in summative rather than diagnostic assessment of classroom skills?
  - develop skills in moderating their assessments in the light of what may be deemed reasonable competence in a beginning teacher? 'After all, the competences in Circular 9/92 provide an agenda for lifelong development!'

- Is it appropriate to divide the assessment of a beginning teacher's competence so sharply between classroom skills (mentor's responsibility) and some more theoretical written tasks (tutors in higher education's responsibility)? Have we not been busy in the last decade trying to produce greater integration between theory and practice? Should this not be reflected in assessment?
- Should higher education institutions be prepared to give out qualifications knowing that they have only been partially involved in collecting the assessment data?

The Oxford experience has been of real development in the language of the first point, but of little in relation to the second. In relation to classroom teaching, and a number of related dimensions such as attendance and punctuality, which might be grouped as professional attitudes, not just the language of official documentation but day-to-day practice, ensures that decisions with respect to the formative and summative assessment of each beginning teacher are taken jointly by the four professionals working with them: two school-based and two higher education-based. All four have to agree for the outcome to be positive – one dissenting voice may mean failure. Moderation of the judgements taken is provided by the breadth of experience of the higher education tutors. In relation to the production of reflective writing, through short and extended pieces, creative support comes from either source, but assessment has been made by higher education tutors only, although there have been occasional calls for mentor participation. To date these have been resisted on the grounds that they are beyond the reasonable call of duty of a busy teacher.

The development by the DES, from 1989, of the articled teacher route into teaching (Allsop and Hagger, 1993) should have created a setting for experimentation in assessment, particularly in relation to the involvement of teachers in the schools where the articled teachers were spending 80 per cent of their time. Scrutiny of literature for a number of these courses is very disappointing, offering little that is new. In one course, in a Student Handbook which has ten pages of instructions on course assessment requirements, there are only three mentions of the role of teachers, thus (my added emphases):

Work at this stage will be assessed by subject specialist tutors in the university and *by mentors as appropriate.*
Internal examiners for course work include the mentor ....
For practical teaching, members of the *pre-assessment* panel will include the mentor and the headteacher of the school.

In the Mentor Handbook there is no single reference to the role of the mentor in assessment of the articled teacher!

Concluding Remarks

It is possible to discern the emergence of shared language, understandings and practices of partnership between schools and HE institutions within initial teacher education. As years of school effectiveness research have shown, the in-school dimension starts from the headteacher but is then transmitted through professional tutors and mentors to other staff, to governors and to parents. It is possible to identify schools where initial teacher education is seen as just the first phase of professional development. The Secondary Heads Association (1993) emphasizes this in a useful pamphlet:

> A teacher is not trained in a single year. Training and professional development continue throughout a teacher's career. Initial teacher training is precisely that – the start of the process. Many headteachers have welcomed the proposal to base a much larger percentage of trainee teachers' time in school because they believe this will improve the quality of delivery of the PGCE course. The new arrangements offer considerable potential for the integration in a coherent process of initial training, induction and continuing professional development.

They appear to understand notions of partnership much more clearly than the promoters of SCITT when they say, 'In teacher training theory and practice are not separable, whether in higher education institutions or in schools'.

Perhaps, if we are given space to develop mutual understandings of partnership, we are on the way to eliminating the view of one teacher that beginning teachers simply get in the way and that in reality '...we want to get on with our own ways and work' (Back and Booth, 1992).

References

Allsop, T and Hagger, H (1993) 'Lessons from a secondary articled teacher scheme', *Journal of Teacher Development*, 2, 2.

Back, D and Booth, M (1992) 'Commitment to mentoring', in Wilkin, M (ed) *Mentoring in Schools*, London: Kogan Page.

HM Inspectorate (1991) *School-based Initial Teacher Training in England and Wales: a Report by HMI*, London: HMSO.

Leighton, P and Aldrich, R (1988) 'Student experiences of teaching practice 1985–86: a study of professional education', *Education To-day,* 38, 1.

Secondary Heads Association (1993) 'ITT – some practical advice', *SHA Update,* 28.

Chapter 4

Taking Responsibility for the Training Curriculum within the School: The View of a Professional Tutor

Anne Evans

Introduction

In this chapter I would like to share my experiences as a professional tutor working with a team of subject mentors in a secondary partnership school linked with the faculty of education at Cambridge University (Homerton College and the University Department of Education). I hope to show, through one example, how schools today have both authority and autonomy in delivering the initial training curriculum jointly with the training institution (HEI); and how the role of the training institution has changed from one of dominance in the past to one more resembling a facilitating partner.

The last five years mark a considerable shift in the balance of responsibility assumed by the two parties – the school and the training institution – for the provision of initial teacher training (ITT). In the past the programme of teacher training was designed and delivered by the HEI which negotiated with schools opportunities for practice placements. Now schools are team members sharing with the faculty in the implementation of training. However, more recent developments – the publication of new proposals for training by the DfE in 1993, the proposal to set up a Teacher Training Agency (TTA) and the imminent demise of the Council for Accreditation of Teacher Education (CATE) – threaten a disruption of this newly established partnership in favour of schools which wish to assume full responsibility for training: 'The Agency will have a clear duty to promote school involvement in initial teacher training' and will pay '...100% grant direct to all types of school which may use these funds to purchase training and support services as they wish' (DfE, 1993). Clearly if schools are given this degree of purchasing discretion, the HEI would provide a client service and subsequently cease to be a partner. The balance of power within ITT is thus changing dramatically within a single decade.

The model of partnership which has been developed in the faculty at Cambridge has evolved on the basis of a number of implicit principles:

- that schools *complement* the work of the HEI by 'making accessible to student teachers their own different and at least equally important expertise' (Hagger *et al.*, 1993) and vice versa
- that both parties should *contribute equally* to the planning and delivery of training
- that the partnership is based on *mutual respect and trust*
- that the partnership should be *continually reviewed.*

The following sections will show how these partnership principles are working out in practice in one school.

Delivering the ITT Curriculum in the School: an Example of Practice

There are four areas of the training programme for which schools in the Cambridge faculty scheme have taken over responsibility. These are: induction, school-based seminars, the daily subject mentoring of students in the classroom and the so-called 'broader professional experience'. In each of these cases, faculty and school representatives together drew up guidelines which, with the exception of one or two requirements, the schools use at their discretion. In order to explain this more fully, it is necessary to outline the structure of the course and the four categories of staff.

School experience

Each secondary PGCE trainee within the faculty of education in Cambridge is attached to a consortium of schools. Consortia vary in size but generally consist of three schools forming a 'principal cluster' together with three schools forming an 'associate cluster'. The principal cluster schools must be within daily travelling distance of the faculty. They carry the responsibility for inducting and for hosting the trainee in term 1 when two days per week are spent in school. In term 2, all of which is spent in school, most trainees will transfer to an associate cluster school. Others will remain in their base schools. Those who remain in their first school for term two are required to transfer to an associate cluster school for term 3 to gain breadth of experience. This term offers a five-week opportunity for enriched curriculum experiences: the 'broader professional experience'. All clusters offer a range of teaching opportunities between secondary years 7 and 13. My own school is one of two 11–16 comprehensives in a principal cluster, the third member of our cluster being a sixth-form college. The range of experience and subject teaching opportunities available to any student is therefore potentially large if collaboration in training between the schools within linked principal and associate clusters is successful.

The four categories of staff

The PGCE course at Cambridge has four categories of staff: two in the school and two in the faculty.

In the school
i) The professional tutor, who has overall responsibility for the management of all trainees within a school and a shared responsibility for planning across the cluster. The professional tutor prepares the school community to contribute to training. This is a mediating role with responsibility for coordinating the training programme, for identifying strengths and weaknesses within the school and within the programme, and for monitoring standards. The professional tutor leads and speaks on behalf of a team of mentors. Professional tutors are nominated by their schools. The faculty has little influence in the selection of either of the two groups of school staff who contribute to the scheme.

ii) The subject mentor, whose main task is to promote the development of the trainee's knowledge and understanding of classroom practice. The mentor has a specific responsibility to coordinate and plan an appropriate timetable for the trainee which will enable him or her to acquire the skills of teaching within a subject area. The mentor acts as a role model with respect to the general professional ethic of teaching, provides professional and pastoral support and guidance, and monitors trainee progress; and as our course handbook puts it, 'is central to the success, growth and development of the student teacher'.

In the faculty
i) The subject lecturer, as the name suggests, is responsible for developing the trainee's subject teaching skills during the HEI-based days and so shares this task with the mentor in school. The subject lecturer provides advice and support about subject content and competency in subject teaching. She or

he liaises with the link lecturer and with the school with regard to assessment when required.

ii) The link lecturer is attached to a particular principal/associate cluster of schools and thus represents the faculty at cluster planning meetings. The link lecturer liaises with and supports the professional tutors in their management and counselling roles; monitors standards across the schools within the cluster; and negotiates the transfer of trainees within cluster schools.

Term 1

The planning for term 1 takes place during the preceding spring term when cluster professional tutors meet with the link lecturer to discuss availability of subject placements for student attachments. This availability differs annually according to staff departures and responsibilities, special requests, illness and so forth, and the schools within the cluster therefore have to be flexible enough to mix and match placements between them in order to be able to offer a reasonable range of trainee places. By September names have been allocated to cluster placements by the faculty. In this way, the cluster takes the initiative during the first stages of planning and the faculty takes over for final allocations. Once a trainee has been allocated to a cluster of schools, all subsequent moves between schools take place within that cluster and are negotiated between professional tutors within the cluster, who may take advice on the needs of the trainee from subject mentors and from the link lecturer. Even in the recent past, the student's introduction to the school was often casual, unplanned, random, even disregarded, as the following quotation from a recent student evaluation shows:

> I arrived. I sat at the back of the Head of Department's class for a day. Then I taught for the remainder of the fortnight. I didn't meet the headteacher and I felt in the dark about the school as a whole. I experienced one extremely difficult situation which, with hindsight, should never have occurred.

We hope that things are different now. Since they became partners in the delivery of training, it has become possible for schools to run an induction programme that is both purposeful and structured. On the Cambridge course, the school-based induction lasts for eight days. The aim of this period is to provide the student with a general understanding of the school as a working community and this is achieved through a balanced blend of introductions, focused observations and time to explore and to reflect. The guidelines for the induction timetable were drawn up by a joint school/faculty committee of which I was a member. The elements of the programme are not requirements but recommendations, it being recognized that schools vary in their ethos, resources, staff expertise and interests, pupil ability, community involvement and so on (also in the students they will receive) and that these differences must be accommodated. In our induction programme, trainees have opportunities to familiarize themselves with the social context and the culture of the school. They may have the chance to meet and talk with school personnel of all kinds, including those associated with the site, with resources, with school meals and with community education. They could visit primary feeder schools, middle schools and post-16 establishments. They are likely to track a pupil throughout the day, to learn something about the implications of teaching children with special needs within the mainstream curriculum and to observe some subject teaching.

It is part of the professional tutor's role to organize and implement this induction programme. This is no easy task given that under the new cluster arrangements we have 18 students in a relatively small school (750 on roll). The professional tutor has to plan carefully in order to minimize the impact on the school, while maximizing the opportunities for the students. In our case, we chose to plan this period very carefully for exactly the above reasons. First, the three professional tutors of the principal cluster schools created daily subject group visits to the sixth-form college, bringing together (for example) all history students to learn about post-16 education. Meanwhile, of the remaining 12 students, it was arranged that six would spend the day in local primary schools, thus leaving at base a manageable group for other tasks. This induction programme was agreed between cluster professional tutors and subject mentors.

Our trainee teachers receive an induction booklet. This was developed in-house and includes information about codes of conduct and uniform for pupils, about resources, about the catchment area; also maps and the names and telephone numbers of all subject mentors, cluster professional tutors and the link lecturer. It is very much an initial survival guide which when used with the official school prospectus gives the new trainee an immediate overview. I am aware of other local schools who also produce booklets for students but this is neither a requirement, nor at this stage a recommendation from the faculty.

After the induction period, the student spends two days a week in school and three days per week in the faculty. Of the two school-based days, one and a half are spent in subject areas under the guidance of mentors and half a day is spent in a cross-curricular seminar, led by the professional tutor. This is one of the means of integrating the contributions of school and faculty:

the seminars are linked to faculty lectures and resource material is supplied by the faculty. The seminar programme is known in the Cambridge scheme as 'Situations and Themes' and in order to understand the objective of the school seminar it is important to view the programme as a whole. A weekly 'theme' lecture on a central educational issue (eg, special needs) is delivered in the faculty. During the related school-based seminar, the theme is explored in the context of practical school experience – that is, it is contextualized as a 'situation'. The 'situation' seminar is organized and led by the professional tutor or a nominated member of the school staff and is attended by the link lecturer who may contribute to it. There is thus integration of school and faculty at the levels of both topic and personnel, with a shared responsibility for delivery of this core course. I have learned that the more I can involve staff colleagues in taking the lead when their own specialism is the topic of the seminar, the greater the interest and relevance the seminar has for the trainees. This may only be possible if I use my time allocation to cover the coordinator's teaching. However, we feel that it not only gives trainees an up-to-date and practical perspective, but is an opportunity for staff development as well as helping all staff to feel involved in the culture and delivery of ITT. As a direct result of this process we have developed our own additional resources which on occasions have replaced those from the faculty. In the new partnership, we have the opportunity to do this and in turn have offered them for use by the faculty – and so by other schools in the scheme – during following years.

The subject mentor's responsibility in term 1 is to provide a carefully structured introduction to the skills of teaching and so to prepare trainees for a full term placement in term 2. Additionally we try to relate the core 'situations' programme to weekly teaching when this is chronologically possible. Thus subject mentors are made fully aware of the weekly programme so that they can facilitate opportunities for work in these areas. During these one and a half days in the classroom, it is important that we provide the students with a range of experiences which are designed to help their personal learning to progress in a variety of ways. Many students arrive with preconceptions about the type of teacher they intend to become, based on their own school experiences. Teaching is, of course, not about charisma alone, and while many students are anxious to get on with the job and prove themselves in the classroom, they have quite a steep learning curve, especially during term 1.

As role model and guide, the subject mentor is central to the trainee's development. Mentors work closely with subject lecturers and panels of mentors are elected by the clusters to discuss and review the subject-teaching elements of the course with the subject lecturers. These meetings are opportunities for the two parties to develop a shared understanding of both the content and presentation of this part of the PGCE curriculum. Mentors often contribute to faculty subject seminars where opportunities arise. In school they guide students along their curve of learning from October's inexperience to December's preparation for going solo. In term 1 the subject lecturer visits the school regularly, and when there, may both supervise the student and liaise with the mentor in a consultancy capacity, this being a transitional stage in facilitating the development of mentoring.

It is important that the professional tutor and the mentors have a shared sense of direction and pace throughout term 1. We believe that a flexible portfolio of experiences is best built up steadily over many weeks. By supporting the trainees through a gradual planned programme, mentors promote their professional development by demonstrating good practice and by sharing planning and team teaching, rather than by supervising them from the back of the room in the style which many of us will recall from the 1970s or earlier. It is now the norm for mentor and students to be delivering a lesson together, each taking responsibility for different aspects. By the end of term 1 the student is leading and the mentor supporting, rather than the other way round.

Throughout term 1 mentors continue to develop the trainees' observation skills. Observation starts in the induction period, when trainees are required actively to observe a specific aspect of teaching or a child. The more focused the observation, the greater the depth of understanding the student is likely to gain and the more purposeful and useful will be the ensuing discussion. Useful focused observation has been done by students helping children with specific difficulties, when acting as learning support assistants. Equally important is students' observation of difficult classroom management situations and the ways in which experienced teachers cope with these. The student previously quoted with reference to induction needed to observe how an experienced teacher would cope with a confrontation situation before being faced with one himself in the classroom. Difficult classroom situations are part of every competent teacher's working life and students, by seeing how we manage them, realize that little can be taken for granted.

By the end of term 1 the professional tutor and mentors have a responsibility to provide a formative assessment document. This is discussed with the student and is transferred with him or her to the term 2 placement school, where it is used as a basis for planning new experiences.

Term 2

The placements available for term 2 will have been decided by the cluster prior to the academic year, and so no negotiation about transfers is necessary at this stage. There may however be a choice of places within a subject area and this can be a considerable advantage since it enables the professional tutors of the schools concerned to consider trainees' needs and place them accordingly. The formative assessment record will have travelled with the student and in most cases discussions will have taken place between both professional tutors and subject mentors of partner schools. In my experience of ITT there has never been a time when we have known so much about the training of a student and received so full a profile prior to term 2. The original request for a term 1 formative profile came from professional tutors at a faculty planning meeting and was subsequently adopted.

Term 2 is largely concerned with trainees going solo, building upon the collaborative teaching undertaken with their mentors during term 1. Over the term, their teaching commitment increases towards two-thirds of a timetable. The speed with which this occurs depends on the mentor and the student agreeing that the next step should be taken. It is important that the trainee also becomes fully integrated as a member of the staff. Hence emphasis is placed on regular attendance at meetings and extracurricular activities. All trainees are attached to tutor groups and therefore involved in the daily tasks and pastoral implications of form tutor responsibility.

During term 2 there is no recommended faculty seminar but we continue to use this weekly meeting time, at first to discuss generic issues and later for individual tutorials. The subject mentors in our school additionally have protected mentor time each week for planning and evaluation discussions with their trainees.

Under the new scheme, major responsibility for assessment has been transferred to the mentors and professional tutor. The need to write to levels of teaching competence directs mentors towards an analytical style of mentoring and reporting, for which guidance from subject and link lecturers may still be necessary. Assessment takes place at interim and concluding stages of this term, and is recorded on a proforma according to competences. However, discretion is left to schools with regard to authorship. In our school, both professional tutor and mentor complete the documentation in order to maintain an overview and a house-style.

Term 3

The school experience in term 3 is negotiated between mentors, professional tutor and faculty staff. If concern has been expressed over a trainee's level of attainment in term 2, a further period of five weeks in a different school within the same cluster offers a second opportunity to meet the teaching competences more successfully. However, for the majority of students the experience in term 3 is one of subject enrichment over a five-week period. What trainees do during this period varies according to their interests and needs, and what opportunities the school has to offer. But what is clear between faculty and professional tutors is that this is not a conventional second teaching practice. Last year many opportunities were created for students to input and coordinate cross-curricular projects, to join language exchanges and field visits, to design and trial curriculum resources and to take an active role in some teaching projects. The projects were diverse and valuable both to students and schools. Mentors in our school classified term 3 as the 'value-added' dimension and as 'pay-back' for the investment of time by mentors in terms 1 and 2.

Some comments on my own experience as a professional tutor in relation to the implementation in the school of the training curriculum as outlined above follow.

Delivering the ITT Curriculum in the School: Some Principles

It is clear to us that we are part-owners of the Cambridge scheme having been involved in the planning of the course. But joint ownership by schools can only come about when they can reliably implement their share of the training curriculum and this depends upon a number of factors.

Knowing the curriculum of training

It is the responsibility of the professional tutor to be fully acquainted with the training programme and to understand its aims and the ways in which the different parts are integrated; and then to lead mentors through the process of learning about it. Training can be successfully established in the school only if there is a clear commitment to it, and a sense of purpose and direction which is shared by all staff colleagues. This can be achieved if everyone knows what being engaged in training means for them as individuals and for the school as a whole. Dissemination of information from the faculty is crucial to achieving a coordinated programme of professional development for the trainee, both within the school and between the school and the faculty.

In order to operate as a successful training school, whether linked with a faculty or working independently, it is also essential to keep abreast of new training initiatives in general and be able to assess their implications for the school.

Making good use of experience and resources within the school

What resources can the professional tutor draw upon in order to offer a programme of training which is seen as appropriate and useful by the trainees and which is integrated with the course at the HEI? Where there is a history of involvement in ITT in the school, there is a basis of experience and knowledge to build upon. We were fortunate in having a team of colleagues whom the faculty had used in partnership practice prior to Circular 9/92, and we were able to use their experience of training. As a cluster, we had also been involved in the Articled Teacher Scheme (ATS). These experiences made it easier for us to assume a partnership relationship with the faculty. Whether or not there have been these opportunities, it is important that from time to time professional tutors review the availability of resources to support the training programme in order to maintain its quality. Do those colleagues engaged in training need further opportunities to extend their skills, and if so, how can these be provided? It may be that some in-house staff development is possible, or that if schools are grouped together as at Cambridge, they can learn from each other, or that the HEI can offer guidance. It is possible that there are some colleagues who might be able and willing to contribute but are currently not doing so. It is the professional tutor's task to find this out.

Discussions on resources are always finance-dominated. The present limited level of funding can only detract from the quality of training that schools can offer. As a result of involvement in the ATS, we realize how crucial protected time for the mentor is to ensure good planning and target setting. Mentor time carries cost implications and funding will need to reflect these if the training that schools can offer is to be more than the minimum.

Changing the climate of the school

Implicit throughout this chapter has been the 'whole-school' approach to ITT. Fundamental to the concept of a good training school is the involvement of all staff in training, either directly or in a supportive role, and their shared understanding of the aims and objectives of ITT. This will come about if training is a central rather than a bolt-on issue on the staff agenda. We may personally feel a sense of pride in our induction programme within one Cambridgeshire school, but it is clear that it could not have happened without the contributions of many colleagues who came together to provide a rich and varied learning experience for the trainees.

If trainees are to have the maximum learning opportunities in a school there needs to be openness and flexibility between colleagues, and it is part of the professional tutor's task to foster this where possible. During the course of a professional placement, a trainee may work with most if not all of the members of a subject department, and will also meet those in charge of specialist areas. In this way she or he may work across curricular areas and may be 'attached' to a number of different staff. Coordinating these arrangements requires good communications and also careful balancing of the needs of trainees, staff and pupils. There may also be a need for a less planned form of flexibility. Each trainee has individual needs and concerns which are unpredictable, and the professional tutor may have to step in and deal with situations which arise from this. For example during the weekly seminar on generic issues in term 2 last year, one student expressed concern about taking Y8. Then most other students expressed a similar concern about this year group. Together we analysed causes and debated strategies, and I in turn took the issue to the senior management group where we further looked at groupings, staffing and other implications. As a result a major decision was made to involve the students in a cross-curricular project so that this year group might feel special.

Engaging in dialogues

Being responsible for a substantial part of the curriculum of training means that the professional tutor is placed in a mediating role between faculty, cluster, mentors, school and possibly parents and governors. Such a person has to be able to speak on behalf of one party to another and inevitably finds him or herself in decision-making situations which were previously rarely experienced. Last year it was apparent that one of our trainee teachers was uncomfortable in the profession. In the past we would have alerted the faculty and handed over the problem. With the changed climate it was natural for us to assume more responsibility for dealing with the situation ourselves and to work through various strategies (such as tutorials) before involving the faculty in a shared meeting at which it was agreed to counsel the trainee to withdraw.

It is the professional tutor who liaises with the link lecturer about any proposals for amendments to the scheme which the school would like to suggest be introduced; and if parents express anxiety about students being in charge of classes, it may well be the professional tutor who acts to reassure them that the school is aware of the need for careful timetabling and that in 'good' school-based training trainees do not take whole classes until they have reached a reasonable degree of confidence and competence in their own and their mentor's view. In our scheme, professional tutors will be in close contact with the professional tutors in the other schools in the cluster. This is in order to organize the richest training opportunities that they can as a group and to standardize trainees' experience sufficiently for them to transfer between schools at the beginning of term 2 with the minimum disruption to their professional development and personal needs.

Monitoring standards

One of the big problems of school-based training is that the more students are dispersed throughout schools, the more difficult it becomes to monitor the standards of the training provided in those schools and to ensure that trainees receive a comparable training experience. The cluster system has an advantage here since the professional tutors of cluster schools can meet together to devise their own system of monitoring and maintaining standards in their schools, and can draw on the experience and support of the link lecturer who is attached to the cluster as a whole. However this remains a major challenge. The professional tutor is in charge of a team of mentors and will need to review the quality of mentoring that the school is providing. If there are difficulties which cannot be met within the school, the subject lecturers are available for advice and support.

Conclusion

Recent changes in ITT have meant for us a growing sense of sharing in the task of training. We feel empowered, have more understanding of our role and of what is to be attained. Collaboration for us means open discussion, sharing in planning and joint ownership of training in partnership with the faculty and between colleagues in our own and cluster schools. We measure our success through student involvement in our particular school and cluster, the quality of pupils' learning and students' understanding of the practical implications of over-arching educational issues. When students work with mentors to provide our pupils with a quality learning experience, we share a sense of achievement.

This chapter has been about the training offered by a school within the Cambridge faculty scheme. I wish to conclude with a strong expression of commitment to *partnership* in training. Schools are the best places for trainees to learn the skills of classroom practice and it seems right that schools should take responsibility here. What we are less able to offer is the overview gained from research. In our partnership scheme we rely on the faculty to provide the wider view: the background and context of teaching in general and the different ways of teaching a subject in particular. Trainees need this view if they are not to acquire too microcosmic a view of education. Now that schools are sharing the task of training, the role of the faculty seems to be changing. Faculty staff still offer a programme of lectures/seminars/workshops in the college or the university Department of Education, and they visit the school as link lecturers or as subject lecturers. But when they are in the school they are more likely to act as consultants and work with the professional tutor or the mentors than to take such a leading role as they did in the past.

References

DfE (1993) *The Government's Proposals for Reforming Teacher Training*, paras 3.15 and 3.5, London: HMSO.

Faculty of Education, University of Cambridge (1993) *PGCE Course Handbook*.

Hagger, H, Burn, K and McIntyre, D (1993) *The School Mentor Handbook*, London: Kogan Page, p. 9.

Chapter 5

Managing the Beginning Teacher in School

Geoff Rhodes

This chapter has been greatly influenced by my work as a professional tutor in an 11–18 comprehensive school in Oxfordshire. The school itself has been committed to the Internship Scheme developed by Oxford University in collaboration with Oxfordshire secondary schools and the LEA. I therefore make the assumption (which is clearly not universally accepted) that managing beginning teachers in school is in the context of a partnership between schools and a higher education institution (HEI). I also take the term 'beginning teacher' to mean 'student teacher' rather than 'newly qualified teacher'.

The chapter is divided into five main sections, the first of which is a general introduction into the nature and scope of the professional tutor's whole-school management role. Section 2 deals with the responsibility for leading and supporting the team of mentors (subject specialists). The third section discusses the provision of pastoral experiences for beginning teachers and is followed by a section which focuses on managing the whole-school programme, including some brief thoughts on inducting and integrating beginning teachers into school. Finally, the last section makes some concluding remarks on the value of partnership and collaboration between schools and universities.

Introduction

The shift in initial teacher education (ITE) towards a more school-based approach has recognized the potential of experienced teachers and the context of the school itself for helping student teachers to learn how to become competent in the classroom. Yet the acquisition of the varied and complex skills of a good teacher involves much more than practising teaching in classrooms or laboratories. Much can be done to support and complement the work of subject-based mentors so that the experience of student teachers in school is neither narrowing nor a hotch-potch. If the school attachment is to be productive and purposeful for the pupils and the school as a whole, as well as for the student teachers, then arrangements for school-based work ought not to be haphazard. The provision of effective learning opportunities for beginning teachers should be carefully managed by someone who will not only work closely with them, but who will also enable a range of other school colleagues to contribute to a planned and developing programme which is geared to the development of effective professionals who are also reflective practitioners. Beginning teachers should be able to develop their teaching skills in a school which they know well and to which they can make a contribution.

In many schools the clear responsibility for implementing partnership agreements with an HEI is invested in the member of staff nominated to be the professional tutor. This is a considerable responsibility and it will be helpful to all in the partnership scheme if the professional tutor has both status and authority within the school. Working in partnership with an HEI can bring many benefits to a school, but there are many potential costs which need to be taken into account so that staff, governors and parents can feel secure that their interests and the vital needs of the pupils whom they serve will be properly represented and protected. This can be more easily done if the professional tutor is in a senior management position. Certainly if there is to be a genuine and developing partnership with an HEI then the professional tutor must have the confidence and integrity to put forward the school's perspective on all aspects of the partnership scheme from the selection of student teachers to assessment procedures, and from funding to the frequency of visits from HEI tutors.

But if there is a need to promote and protect the interests of the school when collaborating with an HEI, there is also an equally important need for someone with 'clout' to speak up honestly for ITT within the school itself. Clearly student teachers and the school staff who are to work closely with them will rely a great deal on the professional tutor being able to obtain for them the support and resources which they need. It is for example an important responsibility of the professional tutor to ensure that the funding which reaches a school to support its work with student teachers is used appropriately. This may require delicate negotiation with the school's senior management team who may be tempted, when the school is under financial pressure, to use funds from one source to pay for a second development. Student teachers will not be able to take advantage of the many learning opportunities in school unless time is made available for teachers to be released from their normal duties so that they can plan and deliver a coherent scheme.

One way in which the professional tutor can create the right environment for effective learning to take place is to try to help the whole school to become involved in ITT. In a sense, the whole school needs to take on the responsibility of mentoring and it can only do this if everyone understands the nature of the school's partnership scheme with the HEI. Colleagues, who have a lot to contribute to the professional development of beginning teachers, will be unable to do so appropriately unless they can understand the assumptions on which the scheme is built and can see how their own specific contribution fits into the scheme as a whole. If the involvement of a school in ITT is merely the peripheral concern of a few dedicated colleagues, working in their departments in a more or less isolated way, then student teachers are not likely to gain a broad understanding of the complex role of the teacher or a knowledge of how schools operate.

New patterns of school attachment should now make it possible for student teachers to benefit from a longer and far less superficial involvement with a school. Greater continuity will not only encourage teachers to invest even more energy and goodwill into ITT but will also provide the beginning teacher with the opportunity to become more fully involved and integrated into the life of the school, to experience many different aspects of the complex role of the teacher over the cycle of a year and to engage in critical investigation and discussion of whole-school policies and cross-curricular issues. It is more likely that student teachers will get the maximum benefit from such opportunities and be more fully prepared for the professional demands ahead if their experiences are planned and managed rather than piecemeal and haphazard. Consequently, collaboration with the partner university is vital if student teachers are to pursue an integrated course with a complementary programme in both school and university.

Working with Mentors

The school-based programme falls into two parts: a whole-school element managed by the professional tutor (ideally in close collaboration with a colleague in the partner university) and a school department element managed by the mentor, a subject specialist. Supporting individual mentors and leading the school's classroom-related team is an important part of the work of a professional tutor in managing the beginning teacher in school.

Mentors are undoubtedly key people in helping student teachers to acquire basic classroom competence so they should be chosen with care and thought. It is a proper responsibility of the whole-school manager to be closely involved in the selection of mentors or even the most coherent of programmes might come to nothing. In choosing mentors the needs of beginning teachers should be paramount, while taking proper consideration of the imperatives of both the individual department and the school as a whole. Student teachers are very anxious about their status in school and are able to learn most effectively when working closely with a mentor who is sensitive to their position as adult learners and also recognizes that their confidence can be all too easily undermined.

There is some value to be gained in a deliberate policy of rotating the role of mentor within a department to promote greater awareness of the partnership scheme. This ought not to take place, however, until each mentor has had the opportunity to develop sufficient expertise and unless other teachers have both the desire and potential to work successfully with beginning teachers.

Once selected, mentors will operate more effectively with guidance and support. Regular team meetings will enable discussions to take place on such things as relevant papers (produced in collaboration with the partner in the scheme) and on appropriate ways of working with students at different stages of their development or at different times in the cycle of their school attachment. Inexperienced mentors may value a second opinion on the programmes (Hagger *et al.*, 1993) which they devise for every student teacher as they develop. Monitoring of programmes is essential, not only to ensure that student teachers are given opportunities to make progress and are treated equitably when there is more than one in a school at any one time, but also to ensure that pupils are not overexposed to inexperienced or insufficiently supported teachers. It is likely therefore that the professional tutor will ensure that the views of interested parties, not least well-informed year heads, are obtained so that the needs of individuals and groups of pupils can be balanced with those of student teachers.

Effective monitoring of the exposure of groups, however, may not be a straightforward task. Beginning teachers learn best when they have the opportunity to work with pupils in a variety of ways (Hagger *et al.*, 1993): sometimes with the group's usual teacher, sometimes with another student teacher, sometimes fully independently, sometimes observing in a structured way and sometimes teaching. After all, 'a punishing timetable forces students into survival routines and drains the energy they need for careful analysis and appraisal of their experiences' (Stones, 1984).

In schools where partnership agreements are renewed annually it may be wise for the professional tutor to maintain records of previous programmes and refer back to them before decisions are finalized about the appropriateness of groups to work with beginning teachers. There should be as little overlap as possible between departmental programmes and the whole-school programme and the professional tutor should seek to ensure that over the course of the school attachment each student has access to a range of classes and, where possible, a variety of subject specialists.

No matter how much care and thought has gone into the design of a subject-based programme some beginning teachers will inevitably experience problems. Concerned mentors may seek to benefit from the judgement and support of an experienced senior manager. It may become appropriate at such times for the professional tutor to liaise directly with university colleagues on behalf of the school, to either seek extra classroom support or reach a consensus on assessment.

In supporting mentors in their work, a professional tutor can help them to draw a balance between their responsibilities to beginner teachers and to other aspects of a particular department's work so that involvement in initial teacher education is not perceived, by colleagues or parents, to impose unreasonable demands which prevent the current or future needs of pupils from being addressed. It is essential for both the professional tutor and every mentor to be able to draw heavily on the expertise of colleagues by maintaining their goodwill towards the professional development of beginning teachers.

While mentors are well placed to draw up and modify subject-based programmes for student teachers, they may need to call upon a more 'senior' manager to make further arrangements on their behalf outside their own departments. For example, a beginning teacher might be able to overcome a problem with a particular class by observing them closely in different subject areas or by visiting the school's special needs department. Likewise, difficulties with a particular teaching skill might be surmounted by focusing on the approaches of a few teachers in the school who are acknowledged as being skilful in that respect. Such arrangements might be more easily and appropriately made by the whole-school manager, particularly if he or she does have authority, though their purpose is to support the subject-based programme.

Pastoral Attachments

The initial education of teachers would be regarded as being inadequate by the professional as a whole if it did not prepare them for the role of form tutor. It is therefore essential that student teachers gain some insight and experience of this role during the course of their school attachment and the responsibility for not only making the necessary arrangements, but also over-seeing them so that the experience is a valuable one, must surely be within the remit of the professional tutor.

To say that experience of pastoral work is essential is not to say that student teachers ought to be given responsibility for form tutoring as soon as they arrive in school. Indeed the opportunity for a longer period of involvement with a single school could provide the encouragement not to rush head-long into this aspect of ITT. Many beginning teachers are even more anxious about form tutoring than they are about classroom teaching and they are more likely not to be swamped by the demanding task in front of them if they are given some time to feel more familiar and settled in the school and more confident in the classroom, before being given another large set of responsibilities and another set of professional relationships with which to cope.

Moreover, the same conditions which enable beginning teachers to acquire classroom competence will also enable them to learn effectively about tutoring. For example they ought not to be regarded as 'substitute tutors' or placed with tutor groups (forms) which are acknowledged to be especially 'difficult' to handle. Similarly the professional tutor should arrange for them to work alongside a form tutor mentor who understands the need for development and progression through protected practice. It is important not to impose unreasonable expectations on inexperienced colleagues who may be struggling to come to terms with a great deal of unfamiliar demands. If beginning teachers are to learn more than merely how to survive they need to be given responsibility gradually, building on positive experiences. Learning through observing experienced tutors and from discussions with experienced tutors and year heads has a part to play as well as learning through carrying out the role itself.

In making arrangements for student teachers to gain experience of pastoral work the professional tutor will need to consult widely to match each individual with an appropriate mentor, within a supportive year team. Having access to student application forms for the course (supplied by the partner university) can help to get to know their backgrounds and get some initial feel for their interests and needs. It might be wise to remember though that such forms were filled in when the thinking of student teachers was understandably at an early stage of development and experienced practitioners who read them should guard against unconscious prejudice.

One advantage of delaying decisions about pastoral placements until after the student teachers have been in school for a few weeks is that by then they should be informed by the judgements of teachers in the school who have already worked with them, albeit in slightly different contexts. Such information would not only be helpful in matching potential mentors with the most appropriate student teacher but also in briefing them properly about their role. The quality of the support which they are able to give to beginning teachers will be enhanced if mentors are kept informed about developments in other aspects of a student teacher's work, for it can help them to modify plans. For example if a beginning teacher is experiencing unusual difficulties in classroom teaching and is already under some stress, it might be sensible not to add to this by burdening him or her with more pastoral responsibility for the time being.

With beginning teachers now able to spend a long continuous period of time in one school there is the possibility of not restricting an individual beginning teacher to working solely with one mentor and one tutor group. There might, for example, be benefits to be gained by beginning teachers in 11–16 secondary schools from spending part of their attachment working in the lower school and part working with older pupils. This could enable them to gain more familiarity with the pastoral curriculum and a greater awareness of the varying demands of the role of a tutor for pupils of different ages. It must be said however, that many beginning teachers do feel less threatened when working with younger pupils. Moreover, in making arrangements, whole-school managers would want to take into account the common need of pupils, mentors, year heads and beginning teachers for continuity, and the particular need of the latter to learn in a structured way through protected practice.

When beginning teachers are restricted to working with just one mentor there is, however, a risk of cloning and the professional tutor might deliberately try to employ strategies to reduce this risk without creating too much disruption for pupils. For example a beginning teacher might be asked to observe every tutor in a particular year team for a number of sessions before settling down to work closely with the appropriate mentor and tutor group for the remainder of the school attachment. Placing more than one beginning teacher at a time in a year team can also pay dividends. The beginning teachers can not only support each other and learn from sharing experiences, but with the agreement and support of their respective mentors they can also arrange to visit each other's tutor group to focus on different ways of doing things. The whole-school manager might also encourage year heads to use, on occasion, meetings of the year team to highlight different styles and approaches to tutoring.

The whole-school manager could also explain the need to avoid cloning when he or she met with the entire year team, but particularly mentors, prior to the arrival of the student teachers in school. The purpose of the meeting would be to pass on relevant papers, discuss the partnership scheme as a whole and answer questions.

Managing the Whole-School Programme

The professional tutor must clearly play a coordinating and supporting role of some importance, but he or she will also be involved in working closely with the student teachers. He or she will take direct responsibility for organizing the whole-school element of the school-based programme and is likely to be delivering a significant portion of it. Where there is a genuine partnership with an HEI, the professional tutor will not have to design this programme in isolation, but will do so in close collaboration with an HEI tutor. Once the period of transition is over, future modifications might take place not only as a result of joint monitoring and evaluation of the programme, but also in the light of shared experiences and views from all schools within the partnership scheme. In this sense collaboration should not be restricted to an individual school working with an HEI but should embrace the entire network of partners.

Without such collaboration the whole-school programme might emerge as a series of compartmentalized, if useful, items relating to whole-school issues but without any overall coherence or purpose. It should rather be a vital element of a fully integrated course. The Oxford Internship Scheme has for example been developed in close conjunction with local secondary schools. The 'General Programme' is built around three major themes (curriculum and assessment, structures of schooling, and taking account of differences) each of which is studied through topics chosen to exemplify one of them. The school-based element of the 'General Programme' is broadly timed to coincide with university-based sessions while recognizing the need for flexibility in the partner schools.

While the 'shape' of the whole-school programme may well vary in different partnership schemes according to their underlying rationale there is likely to be some commonality. Without being subject-based they will help beginning teachers to function more effectively both in classrooms and in schools by investigating a range of whole-school, cross-curricular and professional development issues using the forum and perspective of the attachment school to stimulate critical thinking.

Some might be more likely to release teachers to contribute to a wide-ranging whole-school programme if it were to be arranged for a number of student teachers rather than one individual. There are in any case enormous benefits for the whole-school programme when there are a number of student teachers in a school at the same time and under the same conditions, for it enables a 'group' to be created. This can more easily move the focus away from subject specialism, while also providing the forum to share different perspectives on such topics as language and learning, race and gender equality, ability and differentiation, and so on. There ought to be sufficient flexibility in the programme for the school to focus on particular aspects of its work about which it feels strongly and on occasion for beginning teachers to determine the agenda.

The whole-school programme should run regularly throughout the school attachment of every student teacher and might be expected to take between one hour and an hour and a half per week. The sessions ought to be formally timetabled so that subject mentors will not make arrangements to use these slots in their own subject-based plans. While arranging for the whole-school programme to take place during the school day might rob mentors of some flexibility in their tasks of providing student teachers with a variety of learning opportunities, it does on the other hand signal the importance of whole-school issues for the professional education of beginning teachers.

There are of course some advantages in running the programme at the end of the school day. It would clearly be less restrictive for mentors and, since there would be no financial implications for 'covering' classes, it would be easier for the professional tutor to invite a range of school 'experts' to participate. Schools will rightly weigh up the costs and benefits for themselves, but there is a real possibility that student teachers will not be fully engaged at the end of a frenetic day in school.

The whole-school programme is more likely to be effective if the content, method of teaching and learning and those who take responsibility for delivering it, are varied. As a senior manager with a broad knowledge of the school, its culture and policies, the professional tutor is not only well placed to be a major contributor, but also to arrange for other school personnel (teachers, governors, parents or pupils) to be involved in the programme. For example, the head of the sixth form might be invited to talk about 16–19 provision in the school. Presentations followed by discussion can play an instructive part, particularly if visiting speakers are given some guidance and if the student teachers have been asked to consider the issue in advance of the meeting; perhaps by being given some stimulus material to study. It might though be counter-productive for all sessions to be in this form and other possibilities could be exploited. A mini-bus tour of the school's catchment area, organized soon after the student teachers' attachment to the school, might be very worthwhile. Similarly their expertise as tutors might be sharpened by simulating some active tutorial work which they can later adapt for use in their own tutor groups. The professional tutor might also set up a role play of a parents' evening in conjunction with the schools' parent governors to explore the mechanics of the meeting and how the different participants feel about them. Other sessions might take the form of student teachers reporting back on small investigative tasks focusing on their own experiences or perceptions with regard to a particular issue. Such investigations might also be the basis of any written assignments that might be required during the course as a whole. Written assignments however may not be a major responsibility of the professional tutor. The expertise for setting and marking this aspect of the course might more appropriately lie with a tutor in the partner HEI. The professional tutor's knowledge of the school and contacts within it would though be invaluable in providing student teachers with the means to complete the assignments. He or she could only do this in a planned way if there were close collaboration between the professional tutor and an HEI tutor who shared the responsibility for the whole-school programme. Moreover *ad hoc* assignments or investigations which were rooted in the policies and practices of the school might well prove to be intrusive and too demanding of staff time and would therefore not be in the best interests of the partnership scheme.

It is important to the smooth running of the whole-school programme that clear guidelines should be established from the outset as to how meetings are to function. This is especially relevant when visiting speakers or 'experts' are invited to join the group. A proper balance has to be struck between the professional respect that ought to be shown for the expertise and experience of colleagues (who have voluntarily given up their time) and the need to think objectively and critically. Student teachers have a difficult task in recognizing on the one hand that a school's actions are often pragmatic in the face of many conflicting pressures and constraints, without on the other hand accepting everything which they see with an unquestioning loyalty. The professional tutor may therefore have to adopt the role of apologist on some occasions and devil's advocate on others. Strict confidentiality should apply in all sessions so that uncomfortable views can be voiced at appropriate times and expressed with sensitivity.

One of the first meetings of the whole-school group will be to induct the student teachers into the school where they are to work for some time. As Hagger *et al.* (1993) point out: 'the student teachers' first day in the school is very important, but it should be seen as part of a structured programme aiming to introduce and gradually integrate them into the ethos and workings of the school'. It also provides the opportunity for the professional tutor to make the student teachers feel welcomed as colleagues within the school and to establish the kind of professional and supportive atmosphere that is essential throughout their attachment to the school.

Each individual deserves to feel optimistic that the school, through the professional tutor, will help him or her to develop as a teacher. But it might be best from the outset if the student teachers are encouraged to recognize that working in a busy school will be demanding and perhaps painful at times. It should also be clear however, that the professional tutor's responsibility for meeting the needs and protecting the interests of the student teachers is as great as that for mentors and other colleagues within the school.

The induction process can be made more personal and welcoming by using the information on the student application forms. Certainly a knowledge of individuals' interests can help the professional tutor to integrate student teachers into the school by introducing them to colleagues who are in a position to involve them in the extra-curricular life of the school and make a contribution to it. Integration can be further aided by putting labelled passport photographs onto a staff room notice board to help colleagues put names to faces. More importantly student teachers can be encouraged to mix widely and not just with each other or with fellow subject specialists. However, many colleagues will be more prepared to give their time generously to support new colleagues if they are going to be working in school for lengthy and continuous periods than they might be for transient student teachers whose relatively short teaching practice tends to isolate them in the classrooms of a single department.

Conclusion: The Value of Partnership

There is in schools considerable knowledge, expertise and good will which could be more fully utilized in ITT. While schools have a vital contribution to make to the professional development of beginning teachers, they are more likely to assume a greater responsibility for it if the benefits outweigh the costs and do not detract from their fundamental responsibility to pupils. Working in partnership with an HEI and with other schools to share knowledge and develop a jointly owned scheme would help to reduce the burden on individual schools and lead to important benefits in such related spheres as staff development, induction and appraisal. It would also be the surest means by which schools could discharge their responsibility to future generations of teachers and pupils by contributing to the development of courses of real substance and quality. Genuine collaboration will certainly make the task of professional tutors in managing and learning beginning teachers far less onerous and far more rewarding. Naturally partnership will take some time to develop but it can be built when professionals in both schools and HEIs recognize and value the distinct contributions which each can make.

References

Hagger, H, Burn, K and McIntyre, D (1993) *The School Mentor Handbook*, London: Kogan Page.

Stones, E (1984) *Supervision in Teacher Education*, London: Methuen.

Chapter 6

Classrooms as Learning Environments for Beginning Teachers

Donald McIntyre

The move towards school-based initial teacher education (ITE), with increased resources, responsibility and power being given to school staff, allows the opportunity for a more constructive approach to learning to teach in classrooms. This chapter is concerned with the transfer of responsibility from university to school staff for student teachers' learning in classrooms and with the opportunities which that transfer brings.

The chapter is organized around four general propositions:

1. Classrooms are necessarily the dominant contexts for student teachers' learning.
2. During the years when ITE has been largely based in higher education institutions, there has been little likelihood of classrooms being environments conducive to desirable or efficient learning.
3. A shift towards more school-based ITE creates the opportunity to make classrooms more helpful learning environments.
4. The shift towards more school-based ITE creates *only* an opportunity: no benefits will follow without other necessary steps.

Proposition 1

Classrooms are necessarily the dominant contexts for student teachers' learning

This proposition may seem very obvious now. It was not obvious ten years ago and until very recently an examination of the practice of ITE in this country would not have suggested that it is obvious.

None the less for many years we have had strong grounds for accepting the truth of this proposition. It is persuasively true first as a generalization about what matters to the great majority of student teachers. Learning about what happens in classrooms, about how to make things happen in classrooms, and about what are worthwhile classroom activities is what they care about; and they generally believe that it is through classroom experience that they are most likely to learn these things.

Second, the majority of student teachers are right: classrooms *ought* to be the dominant contexts for student teachers' learning. Especially for one-year courses, preparing people to teach well in classrooms has to be the most important purpose of ITE; and given the context-specific nature of all complex learning, this must mean in large measure learning to address the realities of teaching in specific classrooms.

Proposition 2

During the years when ITE has been largely based in higher education institutions, there has been little likelihood of classrooms being environments conducive to desirable or efficient learning

My suggestion here is that there have been fundamental problems about classroom learning that have been *inherent* in a largely university-based teacher education system. The basic problem has arisen from the fact that one set of people in universities has been responsible for the learning *programme* while another set in the schools has been in control of the main learning *environment*. In these circumstances, student teachers' energies have frequently been focused on the complex but unproductive social task of managing their different masters and mistresses. Four particular problems may be differentiated.

What kind of learning is meant to be happening?

In circumstances where supervising teachers were not involved in the planning of programmes, it was unlikely that they, the student teachers and university tutors would have shared understandings of the kinds of learning that they envisaged occurring in the classrooms.

From the point of view of class teachers, whose responsibility was for their own pupils, the main concern had to be that student teachers should learn how things are done in classrooms, and in their classrooms in particular. In this way, the education of pupils would be minimally disrupted and the student teachers would learn to do things in the ways they are done – which work more or less satisfactorily – in so far as they were personally able to do so. This robust and sensible viewpoint seems to be the one which most teachers have adopted.

From the perspective of university tutors, on the other hand, very different concerns and understandings had to be dominant. Teaching practice was crucial as part of a programme aimed at teaching student teachers how to think about, and to engage with, teaching and learning in classrooms. It was primarily an opportunity to *practise* the use of ideas, strategies and skills which had been read about, explained, discussed and possibly simulated in the university. Otherwise, what was the point of the rest of the programme, into which tutors would generally have invested the fruits of all their own teaching experience, reflection, reading and research?

As pigs in the middle, students teachers had to learn mainly to survive. For the most part, they wisely made common cause with the teachers who controlled the immediate environment and did their best to fit in, learning the necessary conventions, procedures and skills in order to do so. Often they managed to go further, recruiting the help of the teachers in order to impress visiting tutors by putting on performances geared to their preferences. But of course the student teachers generally had their own ideas, based on their own experience of schooling and on selective use of what they had learned elsewhere, including the university. These ideas might sometimes be asserted and they might sometimes be changed by school experience, but more often they would be quietly preserved for later use. Student teachers did of course learn a great deal from teaching practice, but rarely in a planned or conscious way: trial and error learning and having their behaviour shaped by what happened to them, seems the best way of describing most of their learning.

Student teachers' learning was not generally conscious or deliberate, it may be suggested, because *learning* was not the primary goal for them on teaching practice. Meeting the requirements of supervising teachers and visiting tutors and winning the confidence of pupils, or at least gaining control over them, were for most the priority needs. In other words, teaching practice was not mainly for learning, it was for *proving themselves* as teachers: to survive, to 'get through', to persuade themselves and significant others that they could cope with classroom teaching was what it was about. In the absence of shared understandings about the kind of learning that was meant to be happening, this was a very sensible approach.

Problems with the modelling of classroom expertise

One of the best reasons for student teachers spending time in classrooms is that they should have the opportunity to learn from the expertise of experienced teachers. There can be no doubt about the wealth of expertise that is used by experienced teachers on a day-to-day basis; and that expertise ought to be accessible to student teachers so that they can learn from it.

However, where supervising teachers did not have responsibilities as teacher educators, there were major problems with such learning. Student teachers could and did of course learn to adopt the same procedures as their supervising teachers, but the extent to which they learned from their expertise was often very limited and this is reflected in the widespread view among student teachers and supervising teachers that classroom observation had a very limited place in learning to teach, confined to the early weeks of teaching practice. Four specific problems may be identified.

- **The invisibility of skilled performance**: the problem with learning from observation is that you have to understand the skill in what you are observing before you can see it; and without the help of a teacher educator, the novice by definition did not understand, and so did not see, and so did not learn.
- **The practical difficulties of cueing**: modelling is at its most effective for learning when it is *cued modelling*, where significant things to be learned from the performance are clearly pointed out as they happen. Whereas, for example, a driving instructor can give a running commentary on what he or she is doing as he or she does it, this is not generally possible for classroom teachers. Both time and imaginative planning are needed in order to develop cued modelling in relation to teaching.
- **Teachers' difficulties in articulating their expertise**: in the course of their normal working lives, experienced teachers take their expertise for granted and are generally unaware of the sophisticated judgements and decision making in which they routinely engage. Without investing time and thought into the task of teacher education and therefore into reflecting on the nature of teacher expertise, few teachers have either the confidence in their own expertise or the commitment to tease out for the sake of student teachers the complex thinking which underlies their fluent and apparently simple classroom activities.
- **Non-acceptance of teacher models**: left to come to their own conclusions about the teaching they observe, student teachers tend only to see global pictures; and there may well not be a good match between the pic-

tures they see of individual teachers and their own often naïve and idealized conceptions of good teaching. They therefore tend to be very ready to judge experienced teachers as 'not the kind of teacher I want to be' and so to dismiss them as people from whom they have little to learn.

Problems with the practice of classroom skills

Almost everyone would agree that practising teaching in classrooms is an essential element in programmes for learning to teach. But where classroom practice is not planned or controlled by teacher educators, it may not be very conducive to learning. There are two major problems.

- **Teaching, not learning**: an endemic problem for games coaches is that practising is much less satisfying for most players than playing 'real games'. Student teachers, similarly, want to teach, not to practise teaching. And of course, in classrooms pupils are there to be taught, for real. Supervising teachers and student teachers have frequently found it easy to collaborate in approaching the task as one of trying to ensure that the teaching is as good as possible, while neglecting the possibilities of learning from success or from failure. It is tempting to concentrate on being a 'real' teacher, to celebrate successes and to forget perceived failures as quickly as possible, rather than to treat the teaching as practice from which one seeks to learn.

- **The complexity of the task**: even more than with games, learning from engaging in the whole complex task of teaching – as opposed to deliberately practising particular skills or strategies in simplified situations – is very difficult. There is so much happening and so much to attend to when one is responsible for a whole class that it is extremely hard for beginners to focus attention on specific aspects of their teaching which they need to improve. Furthermore, classroom life is so unpredictable for beginners that even if they deliberately try to practise particular aspects of their teaching, such plans can easily be disrupted by unexpected events. Student teachers, even when they do try, cannot easily make classroom teaching fruitful for the practice of teaching.

Problems with feedback on classroom performance

The third main way in which student teachers might be expected to learn in classrooms – complementing modelling and practice – is through getting feedback on their performance. Three particular problems may be identified in getting useful feedback in conventional teaching practice contexts.

- **Establishing a shared frame of reference**: feedback is especially useful when it focuses on aspects of performance which have been agreed upon in advance, when strengths as well as limitations are identified, when the performer's own perceptions are taken into account, when the volume of feedback is not overwhelming and, in general, when it is provided in a very carefully planned, thought out and skilful way. It is especially important for those giving and receiving feedback to have shared expectations about what will be discussed and how, for them to be 'on the same wavelength'. These are quite demanding responsibilities for professional teacher educators and experience suggests that it has been quite unrealistic to expect supervising teachers generally to provide such feedback, when they have no teacher education responsibilities. Not surprisingly, student teachers frequently comment that the most useful feedback they receive is from their visiting tutors.
- **Having situational knowledge**: visiting tutors, however, do not know the characteristics or history of a class or of the individuals within it; nor do they know in any detail about resource or other constraints and possibilities within the school, or about the strengths and weaknesses displayed by student teachers in previous lessons in the days preceding their visits. There are therefore substantial limitations upon the range and quality of the feedback they can provide.
- **Deciding what the feedback is for**: at different stages in a student teacher's development, feedback of very different kinds, and on very different terms, is needed to foster that development. In earlier stages, for example, student teachers need feedback on the adequacy with which they are achieving basic standards in relation to such criteria as pupil attention, interest and comprehension. Later, they need to be able to specify themselves the feedback they require, as they concentrate on learning to take responsibility for the evaluation and development of their own teaching. It is realistic to expect teacher educators to make such distinctions, but not supervising teachers who do not have teacher education responsibilities. Supervising teachers need to be concerned with their own pupils, and the feedback they provide may be designed not to foster the student teachers' learning at all, but rather to look after their pupils' immediate needs.

In summary, then, during the years when ITE has been primarily the responsibility of HEIs, there have been inherent structural anomalies which have prevented coherent planning to make classrooms fruitful learning environments for student teachers.

Proposition 3

A shift towards more school-based ITE creates the opportunity to make classrooms more helpful learning environments

The basic point to be made here is obvious and simple: if the teacher who is in charge of the classroom is also given and accepts the responsibility for being a key *teacher educator* in relation to classroom teaching, quite new opportunities are opened up. In particular, the three basic means of learning already discussed – modelling, practice and feedback – can all be used in deliberate and purposeful ways.

Teacher educator as performer

Where the classroom practitioner is also a teacher educator, valuable opportunities open up for focused and effective modelling.

- **An analytic approach to modelling**: teachers as teacher educators are very well placed to help student teachers focus attention on particular aspects of observed teaching from which they can usefully learn. In particular, they can help student teachers to recognize that they do not need to emulate teachers in their totality in order to learn specific useful skills and strategies from them. An analytic approach to what is happening in the classroom takes attention away from unhelpful concerns with personality types or global styles and attends rather to the tasks which need to be undertaken and to ways of tackling these tasks.
- **Connecting modelling to diagnosis of needs**: teachers as teacher educators are uniquely well placed to identify student teachers' learning needs at particular times. Having identified the aspects of teaching on which individual student teachers need help, teachers can make these aspects of their own teaching especially prominent and visible. Furthermore, they can draw attention to these aspects both in advance and in retrospect, so that student teachers can more easily observe them. It is not of course that one wants student teachers to imitate 'correct' ways of doing things: they each need to develop their own repertoires. What *is* needed however is the demonstration in concrete terms of what it means to achieve, for example, a busy working atmosphere, or clear understand-

ings by pupils of what they have to do, and also the demonstration of some ways in which these things can be achieved. Student teachers frequently need to be offered the beginnings of a repertoire of ways of setting about basic classroom tasks.

- **Making one's teaching more comprehensible to observers**: even experienced teachers when observing one another's teaching tend to recognize only some of the things that are done to achieve desirable ends, and only some of the thinking that has underlain what they observe. Novices recognize very little of what is happening and may well not even be able to ask useful questions about what they have observed. Committed teachers can however, with practice, learn to take their own teaching expertise less for granted and to make explicit to student teachers what they had to do to achieve what may well have looked simple and 'natural', and what they had to take account of in deciding how to do it. At their most sophisticated, classroom practitioners who are also teacher educators can not only reveal the genuine complexity of their teaching but also translate these complex performances convincingly into relatively simple ideas which student teachers will be able fruitfully to assimilate to their own immediate practice.

Teacher-educator as manager of the classroom learning environment

Perhaps the most fundamental shift that becomes possible when teachers accept teacher education responsibilities in their classroom work is that the classroom teaching can be planned to promote simultaneously the learning of the pupils and that of the student teachers. While continuing to give priority to the pupils' needs, the teacher as teacher educator can identify appropriate learning tasks for the student teacher as part of the planned teaching.

- **Collaborative teaching as a context for practice**: normal classroom teaching is too complex to be useful for student teachers' thoughtful practice of specific aspects of teaching at early stages of their courses. On the other hand, attempts to practise aspects of teaching out of context are rarely successful, because of their lack of realism. But teachers who involve student teachers in the planning of lessons and give them carefully chosen and clearly defined responsibilities within these lessons, can create contexts for the practice of teaching tasks which are sufficiently simple and also meaningful parts of whole-class teaching. Carefully planned collaborative teaching is one of the best ways of giving student teachers appropriate practice, and it can only be offered by classroom teachers who are serious teacher educators.

- **Progression in the complexity of tasks**: collaborative teaching can be of many different kinds and is ideal for giving student teachers progressively more challenging tasks as their understanding, competence and confidence increases. In the planning of lessons, student teachers may initially do little more than attend to the teacher's planning but can be increasingly involved until they themselves are doing the planning with the teacher attending to them. Similarly in the teaching itself, the tasks they are given can gradually be increased in scope, number and complexity until the teacher educator's role becomes one of classroom assistant. At that stage, or even earlier, collaborative teaching can become as much a way of enriching pupils' classroom experiences as a means of educating the student teacher.

- **Managing the student teacher's learning experiences**: teachers who are teacher educators have additional advantages to that of having their own classes. In particular, they are members of staff of schools and, in secondary schools, of departments. As such, they have knowledge of other classes and of other teachers and that is knowledge which needs to be used in giving student teachers the learning experiences they need at different times. For example, they need progressively to be given opportunities for teaching more difficult classes, always being faced with challenges which they are capable both of meeting and of using thoughtfully in their learning. There will also be different things to be learned at various stages from observing, or collaborating with, teachers with different teaching repertoires. The teacher educator will need to explain precisely what is needed to his or her colleagues and indeed to recruit them into the acceptance of some teacher education responsibilities; this can be a difficult task. Such sophisticated management of student teachers' classroom learning experiences would, however, be quite impossible for a university-based teacher educator.

Teacher educator as provider of informed feedback

As with modelling and practice, so the teacher as teacher educator is in a position to provide very much better feedback than either a teacher educator who is not school-based or a teacher who is not a teacher educator.

- **Keeping track of the student teacher's learning and experiences**: a teacher educator who knows what a student teacher has done recently – successes and failures, and where he or she has and has not made progress in developing their teaching skills, is well placed to notice events in observed lessons which are relevant to the student's current learning needs. The teacher educator who is in daily contact and conversation with the student teacher and with other teachers who observe or collaborate with him or her can have such up-to-date and extensive knowledge even when she or he, the teacher, observes the student only perhaps once a week. The first priority for effective feedback has to be its relevance to the student teacher's needs and concerns, and teachers who are teacher educators are well placed to provide such relevant feedback. They are also well placed to go one stage further and to collaborate with student teachers in planning the nature and focus of the feedback that will be useful in relation to particular lessons.

- **Using shared knowledge of pupils and their recent learning experiences**: the quality of feedback which a teacher as teacher educator can provide is greatly enhanced by a knowledge of the class, of the individual pupils in it, of their recent lessons, and of the content they have covered previously. The student teacher should also have this knowledge, and so discussion is possible of what classroom events were predictable, what plans were made to anticipate or avoid them, or opportunities that were taken or missed for using knowledge of the pupils to enhance the quality of the teaching. Experienced teachers rely heavily on their knowledge of pupils, but only an observer who knows the pupils can give feedback which reflects this element of teaching.

- **Using shared knowledge of constraints and opportunities**: the practicalities of programme requirements and of constraints of time or resources, for example, are important factors for student teachers to come to terms with. Only a teacher educator who is a teacher within the same context can, however, take account of such practicalities in giving feedback. Recognition of an imaginative solution to problems of lack of time or resources, or questions about why relevant available materials were not used, can add considerably to the quality and realism of the feedback offered.

These then are *some* of the ways in which classroom learning environments can become much improved as a result of the shift towards school-based teacher education. There are certainly many others, some of which will only become apparent as teachers who are teacher educators begin to explore the opportunities open to them.

Proposition 4

The shift towards more school-based ITE creates *only* an opportunity: no benefits will follow without other necessary steps

The tremendous opportunities which have been opened up by a move towards more school-based teacher education, some of which have been outlined, are nothing more than opportunities. Without a high level of commitment, understanding and investment of energies by school teachers, these opportunities will not yield any benefits. Indeed, the research evidence available makes it very clear that a complacent belief on the part of schools that they already know how to do the job will lead to a deterioration in the quality of ITE. It is important, therefore, that we should recognize the conditions necessary for the conversion of the opportunities available into a reality of improved ITE. One major overarching condition has been implicit in this whole chapter:

> **Teachers who have supervised student teachers and who now become 'mentors' have to see themselves as teacher educators and to realize that that is a very different task from anything they have previously done.**

There is a growing body of evidence that teachers and schools are too often inclined to take on the responsibility for ITE without recognizing the scale of the transformation that is necessary. They may be encouraged in this by HEIs which, under political and financial pressure, are anxious to involve schools in their schemes and to suggest that mentoring will be easy.

Among the specific conditions that are necessary, if proper use is to be made of the new opportunities, are the following.

- **Resources and especially time for mentoring**: the available opportunities depend upon mentors being real practising teachers, but also upon their having a substantial amount of protected time for working with student teachers. Schools and especially teachers other than mentors should be far more honest than they generally are about the extent to which student teachers in the latter half of their training give them much needed relief from some of their teaching work. But even when that is recognized, extra resources are needed to provide mentors with something like two hours per week of protected time to spend with each student teacher for whom they are responsible; and if pupils are not to suffer, this must be timetabled time, not time in which *ad hoc* cover is provided for classes.

- **Taking advantage of the mentor role**: even in the most helpful of circumstances, conscientious mentors will always feel that they need more time to do the job better. That being so, it is important that they should use their time effectively, doing those things which their positions make them uniquely well placed to do. The opportunities which have been outlined in this chapter are opportunities open only to school-based teacher educators and it is on using such opportunities that mentors need to concentrate. There are many tasks in teacher education which mentors are *not* generally well placed to undertake, including for example those which involve library study, knowledge of recent research, comparison of different practices and group discussion among student teachers. There is a continuing need for these tasks to be undertaken and for some teacher educators to be employed in positions which facilitate such work. There is also a need for that work to be closely integrated with the work of mentors. But mentors themselves need to guard against squandering their distinctive opportunities through using their precious time to do things which others are at least as well placed to do.
- **Working in partnership**: mentors and university-based teacher educators are each well placed to make their own distinctive kinds of contribution to ITE. But the value of these different contributions is undermined unless they are clearly interrelated and complementary. Most of the problems of the past have been related to a lack of coherence in ITE, a lack of shared understandings about how people can best learn to teach and a lack of explicitness about who is doing what and why. For mentors to be effective teacher educators, they need to become co-planners of the programmes in which they are working, and to do that effectively they also need to become co-theorists about teacher education. The old problems will remain unless mentors accept such responsibilities for thinking about the nature of teaching expertise and how it can best be developed and how therefore ITE courses should operate.

Teacher educators in schools and universities need to work with coherent shared understandings about:

- what the goals of ITE should be
- the nature of teaching expertise and the processes of learning to teach
- the division of labour between mentors and others
- the coordination of mentors' and others' activities
- how to take account of student teachers' preconceptions
- what kinds of progression are important during the training programme.

- **Involving student teachers in thinking about their own professional education**: as we plan what ought to happen to student teachers,
we need to remember that their learning depends upon how *they* make
sense of what they do. The move towards school-based teacher education
carries with it the real danger of encouraging the simplistic views of
teaching and of learning to teach which many student teachers bring with
them. Teaching is *not* just knowing the subject to be taught, having an
appropriate personality and showing commonsense, but the process of
learning this can be slow, confused, painful and unproductive. If student
teachers are to be able to take full advantage of the different kinds of
learning opportunities which mentors and others can give them, they
need help in thinking about what teaching expertise involves and in
learning how to learn to teach. The move towards school-based ITE will
provide few benefits unless student teachers are themselves helped to
think in some depth about the process of learning to teach.

Note

An earlier version of this chapter was presented at the 1993 annual conference of the education section of the British Psychological Society.

Chapter 7

Supporting the Student Teacher in the Classroom

Sarah Tann

A central component of any professional preparation are the periods of practical experience available for trainees. In the case of teacher education, student teachers develop their professional and personal skills in a classroom situation which is as close to the real-life conditions as possible. Such opportunities are now being increased by government regulations which have greatly extended the percentage of time which students are required to spend in school compared to the time they have on HEI-based studies. This change in the balance of the course has intensified the debate about the nature of such practical experience and type of support students require during these periods in the classroom.

All too often decisions about such key professional aspects of training are taken on the basis of institutional, economic or political priorities. Conversely, these decisions might focus on the students' needs: what it is they expect, how they perceive their own needs, what they believe is in their own best interests. This approach reveals a more realistic understanding of the support which would be of most value during their periods of classroom experience. This is not to argue that the 'consumer' (student) is always right. We can also weigh such novice self-analysis against the vantage point of those with a wider perspective of current conditions and imminent changes (tutors) as well as those with greater experience who may be regarded as the 'providers' (teachers). The following discussion is an account of a research project which investigates student teachers' supervisory and mentoring needs.

Background to the Project

The empirical evidence used in this analysis derives from a small-scale project which involved 60 students on their first full experience of classroom teaching over a period of six weeks. Data were collected by an open-ended questionnaire regarding students' expectations of and responses to support provided by both their classroom teacher and local HEI tutor. Tape recordings of a debrief conducted between student and teacher and another between student and tutor were also analysed. Follow-up interviews with a sample of students at the end of the school experience were also conducted. The data from these sources form the basis of the following comments.

In general, the data confirmed other findings relating to students' fears, concerns and needs (Zeichner and Teitlebaum, 1982): fears for their own survival regarding control and discipline, concerns about planning and organization and their need for considerable reassurance and practical guidance. The data also reveal a difference in substance and style between tutors and teachers in their response to student needs.

Although there were marked and generalizable differences between tutors and teachers this distinction was blurred in two ways. First, the difference had been reduced in instances where teachers had previous links with the local teacher education institution. These links included a range of contacts. Some teachers had received their own initial teacher education qualifications from the local institution, others had attended in-service courses there, had participated in induction courses relating to supervision or course development and some had also been involved with student recruitment interviews. By any of these means local teachers had been imbued with some of the same philosophy with which the tutors operated. This therefore reduced the differences which might have been expected to exist between teachers and tutors. However, it was also evident that teachers more recently entering into partnership with the local institution were less likely to have experienced any of these links. This problem was not helped by the increasing work loads on both tutors and teachers who were unable to take on additional commitments and was further exacerbated by cut-backs in opportunities and financial support for joint meetings and consultations.

The second reason why the school–institution differences were blurred was a variation between HEI tutors in their familiarity with and knowledge of the course. The tutorial team contained some part-time staff newly brought in to help with supervision. There were also some full-time staff who were not accustomed to school supervision. Hence the tutor's familiarity with the particular course and with higher education in general was often an important factor which appeared to affect their supervision style. Again, the need was evident for increasing opportunities for close contacts, careful induction and continuous planning with review between all those responsible for initial teacher preparation so that support could be harmonized. However, such opportunities for dialogue between tutors were also being reduced in the same way as those between tutors and teachers.

Main Findings of the Questionnaires and Debriefs

There are four areas of student concern which elicited different responses from teachers and tutors.

Students' needs

In the early stages of their school experience students expressed needs which were survival-orientated and person-orientated. The most frequent statements were those seeking encouragement and confidence-boosting through help and practical advice. In particular students wanted tips to solve the problems they believed they were experiencing. In the first instance, these were commonly identified as classroom management. They also wanted specific advice on individual tasks and pupils. This need was most often couched in terms of discipline. Further, students wanted to be liked by the pupils and were thus concerned with establishing friendly relationships sometimes at the expense of a 'teacherly' presence.

The students' perception of their needs quickly became a 'teacher-orientated' response to the situation: wanting to be 'in charge' so that the lesson would 'go well'. They wanted a boost to their confidence in their ability 'to manage' which they saw as being the first prerequisite of 'becoming a teacher'. But to 'make them [the pupils] learn' was sometimes reduced to a discipline battle and students perceived their need as one of wanting the authority to impose rules and sanctions. Such manipulation of extrinsic motivation to learn was seen by the tutors as a 'negative' perception of pupil problems leading to inappropriate student solutions. The response by tutors was usually to try to adopt a more 'positive' approach by redefining the problem in terms of task appropriateness. Specifically, tutors encouraged students to review their lesson and to elicit, by questioning, some evidence of the intended learning objectives of the task or activity. This was in order to encourage the students to reassess the suitability of the task in relation to the abilities and interests of the pupils: they were required to make their own assessment of such aspects as match, progression, motivation and worthwhileness. This appears to have been perceived by the tutors as being a way of helping the students, by reconceptualizing both the problem (which students had defined as one of management) and the solution (which students had seen as the need for new strategies to meet the requirements for control).

Such a shift required the students to move from a concern with themselves as teachers to a more 'learner-orientated' approach to the problem. This meant they needed to consider ways of enhancing intrinsic motivation for learning which, it was hoped, would reduce the need for external controls. However, the questioning style used by many tutors was frequently experienced by the students as additional stress, because they felt it to be a form of 'testing' rather than active construction of their own solutions. Further, while the tutor could help the students re-examine their planning, they were not in a position to help the students with detailed knowledge about the abilities of the children so that a better match could be made, which is what the students believed they needed.

Teachers, by contrast, tended to respond to student concerns for survival and management help by giving concrete advice in terms of existing classroom routines and practices which the children already knew and, therefore, to which they were likely to respond quickly. Teachers also made suggestions about task appropriateness. This was usually in terms of specific children's abilities and interests. Such practical 'technical-instrumental' information was perceived by the students as immediately meeting their needs. Where such advice was seen to be likely 'to work well' it boosted student confidence and also their sense of security within the classroom. In these areas, teachers provided a closer match with the students' perceived needs and their short-term requirements than did the tutors.

Professional orientation

The second most frequently expressed area of concern which differentiated tutors' responses from teachers' responses was the student's own development as a teacher in the classroom. Students voiced their anxieties about their performance: 'How well do you think I'm doing?'; 'What should I do next?' The feedback received on these vital questions was often described by students as inadequate in terms of specificity. The content was characterized as being bland and nebulous so that the student could read whatever they liked into a comment. Or, it was perceived as being sharp and overly critical. These differences often appeared to relate to the medium by which the feedback was offered, whether oral or written.

The differences between oral and written comments stimulated several responses from the students. For instance what was said was sometimes perceived by the students as being at odds with what was written. Oral comments were often gently encouraging and written ones appeared negative. (Alternative suggestions were perceived, by a few, as veiled criticisms and therefore also as 'negative'.) Teachers and tutors, however, often used the two different media for distinct purposes and for different time-scales. Oral comments were indeed intended to be generally sympathetic and supportive in order to boost confidence in the short-term. Many tutors and teachers used the written comments to focus on the specific, in the belief that specifics needed to be remembered if they were to be helpful and a written record acted as an *aide mémoire* and would be of benefit in the medium- and long-term.

Teachers were often reluctant to make written comments but where they did this varied between general remarks relating to developments or problems occurring over the whole week or a focus on a very specific incident. However, tutors generally made a written report after each visit relating to that specific session which they had seen. Written comments were generally perceived by the tutors as a summary of what had been discussed and 'agreed' between student and tutor during the debrief. They might offer a number of different kinds of suggestions: those which focused on the pupils relating to the learning processes and on the content of the lesson: what strategies might help to avoid similar future problems, which alternative activities might have been more appropriate, or how to extend the work already begun. In addition, suggestions might focus more on the student and relate more particularly to ways in which they could try to broaden their own professional repertoire and deepen their own analysis. For example, a student who was now confidently planning and managing two groups could be encouraged to take the whole class for limited periods. Or, a student who was confident in a teacher-controlled learning context could be encouraged to try to introduce more learner-controlled activities. Or, students might be helped to collect data more systematically rather than rely on selective impressions. This would allow them to examine the fine grain of a particular classroom strategy so that it could be more closely reviewed, reflected upon and refined.

Another difficulty incurred in the method of feedback was its timing. Immediately after a classroom session the student was likely to be in an emotional state, whether on a high or a low. What was needed then and there, in an oral mode, was often very different to what might be needed some time later, which was reflected in the written mode. Also, the memory of the oral mode may well be inaccurate and seem to create further tension between the two sources of feedback. Tutors were always in the position of having to give feedback immediately, in this sometimes rather emotional period. However, teachers, because they were available for comment daily, were often in a better position to delay, adapt, modify and extend their feedback to suit the changing needs of the student as they reflected on what transpired earlier, how they felt about it then as well as later. The teacher was also available sometime afterwards when the student might want to raise new points.

A further differential between tutor and teacher was the style of feedback. Teachers frequently made specific suggestions about prospective additional follow-up activities, or gave retrospective ideas for alternative tasks which might have been more suitable, or corrective guidance on teaching strategies which could have been usefully employed at that time but which could also be tried on subsequent occasions.

However, the style of many tutors was markedly different. It tended to focus on eliciting strategies which were designed to encourage introspective analysis on the part of the student, so that they engaged in self-analysis regarding what they were trying to achieve, why, how and in what respect they were successful. The questioning (sometimes very Platonic in the way they led a student to a particular conclusion!) aimed to help the students find their own solutions and to feel that they could be responsible for their own learning and in fact that they had the knowledge available to help themselves once this had been brought to light by a 'critical friend' (Zeichner and Tabachnik, 1982). This was also intended to boost confidence as well as greater professional independence. In some situations students became frustrated and wanted 'to be told'. Others felt a loss of confidence as they realized how much more they needed to know. Still others were excited at the challenge and their self-esteem enhanced when they did in fact feel that, had they thought a bit more first, they knew it all along.

Student files and assessment

The third recurring area of concern related to the ubiquitous student file and the harsh realities of assessment. In this respect students sought reassurance on the layout of their file, its appropriateness of style and adequacy of content. Students asked 'Are my lesson plans OK?'; 'Do I have to do all the objectives every time?'; 'How much do I have to write for evaluations?'; 'The record keeping is in my head mostly.'

On this issue the tutors usually had a lot to say! But students often found that advice differed between tutors and seem to be dominated by the personality and preconceptions of the individual tutor: it became a very 'tutor-orientated' issue. This had the effect of often increasing student fears and of reducing their confidence and sense of security.

Concern was also expressed about the students' need for feedback on their progress: 'Will I pass?'; 'Is this what you want?'; 'Did it go well?' Here again the views of teachers and tutors often varied. This was sometimes because teachers and tutors observed different sessions during which students performed in markedly different ways. However, there were also differences between the teachers and tutors in terms of their expectations concerning the speed with which students progressed and the level at which the students operated. This was particularly so with regard to moving from group to whole-class control, or the degree of competence expected in record keeping, detailed planning or noise and movement tolerance.

In this area of file and assessment, the teachers' comments were often believed to be of more short-term practical application (daily). The tutors' comments were regarded as being of greater significance in the medium-term (termly module) because it was felt that in the last resort it was the local institution which set the mark. Thus it became a 'college-orientated' issue.

Long-term reflections

A final concern which the students (less frequently) raised concerned a need to 'know more' about what makes children tick, how to motivate them and how to recognize different preferences in learning styles so that the student could match these better. In these cases, students were often more confident and were no longer concerned with personal survival. They believed that they had learnt to analyse learner needs and to respond with a growing repertoire of tasks, contexts and teaching strategies which were beginning to meet the needs of differentiation and of progression. In this respect they felt that they were 'managing' competently.

They now wished to deepen their understandings and to develop practical theoretical frameworks to guide their further growth. These students demonstrated a professional and long-term concern with a deeper level of understanding which went beyond the specific situation in which they now found themselves. Instead they wanted to build up generalizable frameworks of understanding which embraced increasingly fundamental and basic concepts of the 'hows', 'whys' and 'with what effects' of learning and teaching which could be transferred to other classroom situations in which they worked later.

Such requests for support showed that the students were becoming aware of their own personal professional growth which they were developing through critical reflection. These students were ones who welcomed the tutors' contribution in particular. This was partly due to the eliciting style of feedback which the tutors tended to use which encouraged the students to actively engage in constructing their own understandings. Also the substance of the tutor's feedback was more likely to help students link their own emerging private theories into existing public theories. In this way tutors could offer a distinctive contribution which helped students develop strategies which could be generalized beyond the immediate classroom situation and would therefore be valuable in other professional contexts which the students would encounter during their initial training and subsequent career.

Summary and Conclusions

Initially, most of the students' needs were expressed as a desire for short-term tips and teaching strategies and were characterized as being situation-specific. This was typical of the substance of the teachers' responses. For this reason teachers were often seen as being more immediately 'useful' than tutors. Students clearly felt very emotional and often vulnerable in the classroom situation. Their comments reflected considerable personal angst. In such a state, they welcomed the fact that the teachers adopted a 'telling' style of feedback and gave practical advice which boosted an immediate sense of security.

Understandably students were initially survival-orientated and expressed 'personal' concerns. Later, after gaining confidence with practical aspects of classroom management, their needs were more pedagogically-orientated and showed concern for the pupils as learners and the teachers' role in developing learning experiences. Later still, those who had already developed some measure of confidence in the classroom moved beyond the specific situation and became more professionally-orientated. They became aware of the contexts within which they were operating and of the wider consequences of their actions. They became excited and challenged by being asked to draw upon and to generate generalizable frameworks. They welcomed the integration of theory with practice as it helped to 'make sense' of the specific situations in which they found themselves. Such students enjoyed the opportunity to try out their own emerging personal theories deriving from their experiences in a professional context. These needs were more closely met by the tutors' responses. In contrast to the teachers, tutors adopted an 'asking' style and tried to elicit and probe to promote rational self-analysis. This was done with the purpose of providing long-term stratagems for professional development. Thus it would seem that the differentiation in tutor and teacher responses to changing students' needs at different stages was crucial.

However, the demands of the file and of the forms of assessment seem to detract from the emerging professional-orientated needs of some of the students. These demands were 'college-orientated' and tutor-specific and caused considerable anxiety. The file sometimes appeared to fail to contribute to the process of helping to meet student needs for personal confidence and security through recording practical tips or from the pedagogical analysis by guided self-appraisal.

Issues arising from the Findings

Knowledge, skills and contexts

The students were anxious and overwhelmed by how much they felt they needed to know and the seeming enormity of the task. This raises questions about the amount and timing of knowledge to help the students. A teacher education course is inevitably a linear experience. Yet the characteristic of teaching is that it is a complex, multi-faceted activity which combines scientific analysis and professional artistry. All teacher education courses have had identified for them, by the government, the component knowledge and skills which students are expected to acquire in order to become competent entrants to the teaching profession. For secondary courses these are classified under the broad headings of:

Subject Knowledge
Subject Application
Class Management
Assessment and Recording of Pupils' Progress
Further Professional Development.

For primary courses the headings are:

Curriculum Content, Planning and Assessment
  − whole curriculum
  − subject knowledge and application
  − assessment and recording of pupils' progress

Teaching Strategies
- pupils' learning
- teaching strategies and techniques

Further Professional Development

However, although it is possible to enumerate competences in terms of the knowledge and skills expected of teachers at the end of their initial training, it is less easy to decide on the best strategies for inducting students into the holistic realities of the classroom. Is it better to adopt an holistic 'top down' approach and let the students get a general feel of the whole situation before then helping to refine their understandings of the parts and their interrelationships? Or, is it better to adopt a linear 'bottom up' approach and initiate them into selected components before building up to the whole complexity? Or, is it better to focus on the practicalities of the specific situation or to concurrently encourage students to question practice rather than learn to imitate first, question later and then unlearn and relearn?

Choices about these aspects clearly affect the nature of the practical experiences which the students are offered: whether it be a controlled building up of the size of responsibilities (one group, two, half then all the class), or a building up of the time for which students have responsibility for the class (story time, register, one session, a morning, all day), or a building up in the nature of the responsibilities (implementing the class teacher's plan, planning with the teacher, planning alone). For example, where stress is related to the apparently overwhelming complexities of classroom life, students may find it more comfortable to 'practice' in a micro-teaching context. In this way a particular strategy can be isolated and the complexity reduced. However, some students find the idea of video, or of 'teaching' peers, even more intimidating. For these students it may be more helpful to work in a classroom in pairs, or on a day-a-week serial practice. Again for some it is even more demanding to work collaboratively or on a sequence of sessions which destroys the rhythm of classroom life. While the debate about holistic and linear approaches may continue, most courses adopt an holistic spiral approach to the learning process. This assumes that all of these skills and areas of knowledge are necessary all of the time and that they will become refined and developed through being revisited at each period of practical school experience.

Substance, style and sources of support

Although student needs can be identified and possible stages suggested, the duration of each stage for every student is impossible to predict. If a spiral approach to student preparation is adopted and the need for survival, pedagogical and professional development accepted as necessary for initial training then it would seem important that the distinctive inputs from teachers and tutors are concurrent. This would offer greater opportunities for the significance of the contributions to be harmoniously integrated into an holistic professional practice. For example, acquiring competence to deal with everyday incidents in the classroom through the application of pre-given tactics suggested by the teacher should not be divorced from also questioning why it works and what the student means by 'works'. Such questioning encourages the articulation of goals and objectives in the short- and long-term. Similarly, when students are trying to generate personal theories to underpin their own actions, this needs to be promoted through interaction with tutors as well as teachers and peers in order to support the student in becoming professionally-orientated.

Apart from the holistic nature of the professional role, a key area of concern which was clearly evident in the questionnaires and interviews was that of the emotional and stressful nature of the students' experience. It was stressful because of their own personal insecurities about 'being successful' and professional inadequacies which meant they felt lost and 'didn't know enough'. Support for the students also needs to address these factors.

The findings of this research indicate that some students found tips gave them instant initial security. Later, the eliciting process, which encouraged self-appraisal, was found to increase the confidence of others. This was because it helped them to pinpoint their progress (so that they felt they could recognize their development) and to clarify any problems (so that they might appear easier to grasp). Such self-appraisal was achieved through analysis, critical reflection, on-going stock-taking and target-setting. A further way of alleviating this stress and shortening the 'survival' stage could be by altering the kind of evidence students use to evaluate themselves. Because of the emotional and stressed nature of the experience, student evidence is often very unreliable; it may be impressionistic, incomplete or inaccurate.

For evidence to be a sound basis for self-appraisal it is better if it is descriptive (rather than judgemental), dispassionate (rather than charged), discerning and discriminating (rather than generalized), diagnostic and forward-looking. Systematically collected evidence could serve to pinpoint the problem. This could clarify an otherwise cloudy situation and reduce the problem to more accurate proportions. In turn, this might boost self-esteem and develop a sense of being able to define a problem, analyse it and proceed to solve it, which in the long-term could perhaps promote greater professional self-sufficiency.

Initially, both tutors and teachers could help to collect such evidence on behalf of the student and discuss with the student what would be of most value. Thus the student can exercise control of the criteria in the process of appraisal and the supervisors will be working for the student rather than setting up their own criteria and appearing to pass judgements on the student. For example, a student might be concerned about their introduction or instructions at the beginning of a lesson, or the way they conduct a class discussion. In such a case a supervisor could note down the structure of the information given, the nature of examples given, the clarity of signposts and of section summaries, or tally the opportunities for pupils to contribute and occasions when pupil understanding was checked. Similarly, a supervisor could tally the types of questions asked in a discussion, the distribution of questions amongst members of the class and encouragement given to pupils to respond to each other and not always through the teacher.

The roles of tutor and teacher: duplicative, integral or contradictory?

The evidence so far leads to a number of basic questions which need to be answered. Is it appropriate that the training of students should be principally in the hands of classroom teachers who appear to be better able to meet the initial needs of the students? If training becomes entirely school-based might students be limited to only one kind of support which may not fully meet their needs? Can we expect teachers to change their kinds of support to include the extended 'tutorial' role, given the increasing demands already being made of them? Should tutors be included in the training process so as to continue to make their distinctive contribution?

It would seem that in the classroom situation students gradually learn to differentiate tasks and responses to suit the different needs of pupils. So, too, do students need differentiated responses from their supervisors. Such differentiation is difficult to achieve without knowing the individual student well and having been involved in their development and progress over a lengthy period of time. Thus closer cooperation between school and local training institution is desperately needed. But current circumstances seem to make such a goal ever more difficult to achieve for lack of time, opportunity and money.

These circumstances also make it very difficult to provide the support for the teachers and tutors which they also require to help to prepare them for this particular aspect of their work (Zeichner and Liston, 1987). Classroom teachers are not experts on articulating pedagogic principles and supporting students; neither are tutors' subject specialities all that is required to support pedagogic action in the classroom. Further, both kinds of supervisors need to understand each other's role better so that each can play a constructive and complementary part. It would seem from an examination of student perspectives on their periods of classroom experience that indeed a close review is appropriate. However, it is not just the relocation of greater parts of their professional preparation from local training institution to schools which needs to be examined but also the nature, style and sources of support.

An element of student insecurity and stress is possibly inevitable. But professional initiation doesn't need to be a trial by ordeal. It perhaps needs to be staged with different locations, experiences, periods and support at different times in the course of professional development. The greatest distortion of the profession is perhaps to examine initial preparation without seeing it within the context of a whole pattern of long-term professional development and renewal for pre-service and in-service. But that's another story.

References

Zeichner, K and Liston, D P (1987) 'Teaching student teachers to reflect', *Harvard Education Review*, 57, 1.

Zeichner, K and Tabachnik, R (1982) 'The belief system of university supervisors in an elementary student-teacher programme', *Journal of Education for Teaching*, 8, 1.

Zeichner, K and Teitlebaum, K (1982) 'Personalised and enquiry-oriented teacher education', *Journal of Education for Teaching*, 8, 2.

Chapter 8

The Influence of Tutors and Mentors upon Primary Student Teachers' Classroom Practice

David McNamara

Introduction

The major part of the emerging corpus of theory and research on school-based mentoring examines mentoring within its social and educational circumstances and with reference to policy and quality assurance issues; it also describes emerging practices and makes proposals for what is regarded as 'good' practice. Apart from a few studies, investigations have paid too little attention to considering whether and to what extent the information, advice and support which it is assumed mentors and tutors provide actually informs student teachers' preparation for practice and subsequent teaching. Debates about how student teachers' mentors and tutors may contribute to initial teacher training will be better informed if they bear in mind evidence which describes how student teachers actually develop their professional capability in school-based settings.

The Hull Study

The essence of the research programme was to investigate primary student teachers' teaching performances within the classroom and to assess the manner in which advice and contributions from class teachers (mentors) and university education tutors (tutors) informed and influenced the ways in which the students prepared for and carried out their teaching. The research was undertaken with primary students pursuing a one-year postgraduate certificate course (PGCE) at the University of Hull. The course, which focuses training upon the Junior/KS2 phase, is already 50 per cent school-based, with the students spending three periods of from four to six weeks in school, together with one day per week during the university-based part of the course.

It was decided to adopt a research strategy which concentrated the investigations upon a relatively small sample. This is because it was felt that learning to teach is, to a marked degree, an individual and idiosyncratic experience for the student which depends very much upon particular school practice placements with their special mix of children, resources and the 'culture' of the school, and the support and advice offered by individual tutors and mentors. It was judged that worthwhile and informative evidence would be qualitative, rather than quantitative. The sample consisted of 'cases'; a 'case' being the student on a school practice together with his or her tutor and mentor.

In the light of events at the time (the research was undertaken during 1991–3) and the then emerging DfE policies on the future of teacher training, it was decided to select a sample of practice schools which represented the range and quality of experiences which students encounter during periods of school practice.

Information was acquired in two principle ways: semi-structured interviews with students during their periods of school practice, and linked interviews with their mentors and tutors; and classroom observation sessions during which 'critical incidents' in the students' teaching were identified for subsequent discussion with them. The data collection was undertaken by a semi-retired teacher trainer and semi-retired headteacher, both of whom were highly regarded in local schools; they were chosen to ensure effective rapport with members of the sample, both students, tutors and teaching staff.

In concrete terms the main research questions were:

- Who and what determines the material or context in which students teach?
- Who and what determines their teaching methods and the ways in which they teach?
- What particular influences inform students' planning and practical teaching?

The major themes which emerged from the research are addressed below.

Who Decides What is Taught and How it is Taught?

An enduring image often associated with teacher education courses is that the material which student teachers teach during their periods of school practice and their teaching styles and approaches are shaped by the information and advice provided by their tutors and influenced by prevailing educational theories and preferences, modified following discussions with class teachers in their practice schools. It was decided to explore with students and their tutors and mentors how decisions were actually taken about what they should teach and the teaching styles or methods that they should use during their teaching.

Student interviews

Prior to periods of school practice the students were interviewed and, among other things, they were asked what they were going to teach during the practice and then asked who had made the decisions about the material to be taught. They were also asked to comment on the involvement of themselves, their mentor and their tutor in the discussions about what and how to teach and the organization of their school practice timetable.

What to teach
The students' responses were grouped into four broad categories.

- In the significant majority of cases, 17, students reported that, in broad terms, what they taught was determined by the mentor and general school policy but that they were involved in the discussions and given some say in deciding what to teach within the context of what was laid down. In these cases students reported that their tutors were not involved in the decision making.
- In five cases the students reported, as above, that they had some flexibility within requirements set by the mentor and school but that, in addition, their tutor had been asked for advice or been drawn into the discussions about the material taught and the timetable.
- In three cases students reported that what they taught and the organization of the timetable was prescribed by their mentor. Either the mentor or the school had an agreed and fixed curriculum plan and the student was required to fit in.
- Finally, in three cases, students reported that they were given considerable free choice by the mentor in determining what they taught. In one case the student was, in effect, left to 'sink or swim' but in the other two the mentor made it clear that the student could decide what to teach but expected to be consulted and was willing to advise.

The evidence is unequivocal and convincing. The university education department had, as do all teacher training institutions, established certain desiderata for the students' teaching practices by indicating, for example, that students were expected to teach all the class for a nominated proportion of time and to gain experience teaching all areas of the curriculum. Beyond such parameters it is clear that the overwhelming majority of students perceived and reported that they were placed in contexts where, in general terms, what they taught and when they taught was very much determined by their mentor (usually bearing in mind the school's curriculum policy) but that they were involved in discussions and given some flexibility. In only a few cases was the tutor consulted or involved. The *de facto* experience facing most students was the extent to which the mentor (or school) was prepared to involve them in discussions about what to teach and the genuineness of the offer. At best teacher trainers had only a marginal role in influencing what students taught during their teaching practices.

How to teach

The students were, for the most part, placed in situations where they could not decide what they taught, but it did not necessarily follow that they would be similarly constrained in terms of how they taught. They were, therefore, asked about the teaching methods they planned to deploy during their practice and the use of prescribed teaching materials, such as published schemes of work.

In 25 out of the 28 cases students reported that they were given considerable flexibility in terms of deciding how they were to teach and in their choice of methods and approaches. Students tended to use terms such as 'very flexible', 'totally flexible' and 'left to the student'. Indeed mentors usually encouraged students to decide upon their teaching methods for themselves.

In one curriculum area, however, there was an exception. In 16 of these 25 cases students reported that this flexibility had not extended to the teaching of mathematics. The schools had adopted commercially-produced mathematics schemes which were closely followed by all classes. Students were required to ensure that children worked through the mathematics scheme at their own pace during designated lessons each week. Most students were offered the opportunity to teach extra mathematics and to do so using their own methods, usually as an adjunct to topic work or science, but they still had to cover the scheme.

In two cases students reported that there was no flexibility or very little and they were required to fit in with their mentor's approach. In one other case flexibility did not exist in that the student had simply decided to 'go along' with the teacher's routines and methods.

Tutor interviews

What to teach

The ten tutors who supervised the sample students during their school practices were asked to what extent they felt that the content of students' schemes of work and lesson plans had been influenced by their suggestions and to what extent by the mentor and school. All tutors, except for one, were quite clear that the basic content was influenced by or specified by the mentor, usually in the light of school curriculum policy. They felt that once the content had been nominated by the mentor then, subsequently, they or other tutors (such as subject specialists) could have some influence upon students' decisions about the detail and ways in which specified content could be taught. The tenor of their replies is indicated by the following, for example (all quotations are from investigators' interview records):

> Content was identified by the teacher initially and in some cases content was included because of SATs requirements and in order to plug gaps which the teacher had not covered. Tutors' influence came at the next stage when she helped students design the structure and tease out the working pattern.
>
> Broad content is dictated by school and staff; influenced greatly by individual class teachers. However, there are some signs of curriculum tutors' suggestions and ideas being used.

How to teach

For teaching methods, tutors were asked two focused questions, since it was felt that their analysis of methods and materials could be detailed and extensive.

First they were asked whether they had any say in how students should organize and arrange their classrooms. Half the tutors, five, felt that they had no say or very little in deciding how students organized the classroom. Moreover, they felt that it was usually preferable for the students' practice that they should fit in with existing arrangements. For example:

> No ... this open plan school is bursting at the seams and there is no flexibility, it would have been beyond possibility for anyone to intervene.
>
> Teacher likes her own way of organizing.

Three tutors felt that they could have some influence upon how the class was organized, especially where they had decided that it was necessary to intervene in the interests of effective teaching. For instance:

> Good classroom management was being hindered until my suggestion to remove large centre-piece display to side of room. In most cases I've not seen the need to change much of existing organization.

> I suggested alterations to seating/furniture to help student struggling with class control, but I do like to discuss with the class teacher.

Second, tutors were also asked whether they thought that they shaped or informed students' specific teaching performance or skills in any way. A few tutors wondered how enduring their influence upon students' specific teaching skills might be but all of them were able to cite instances where they felt that their particular advice or interventions had had a demonstrable effect upon students' teaching. For example:

> Her style was originally inappropriate for the age-range she was teaching. Over the period of the practice, by regularly reminding her of this, I was able to achieve a change.

> An early PE lesson I saw was more of an organized playtime than a movement lesson. My advice was to go for quality of movement and a link between music and movement. She followed this successfully.

Mentor interviews

The mentors were asked to what extent they felt that it was the school's responsibility to determine what was taught and how it was taught.

In every case the mentors said that it was theirs and the school's responsibility to determine what was taught and, to a lesser extent, how it should be taught. The only differences between them related to the extent to which they felt that there could be any discussion or negotiation with students or their tutors. Some teachers were adamant that there was no scope for discussion while others felt that there should be a partnership with as much flexibility as possible within the current context in which primary schools are working. There was one overwhelming factor that determined the mentors' responses and the insistence of the majority that they should have the deciding voice in students' teaching. This was the circumstances brought about by the introduction of the National Curriculum and the requirement to comply with the programmes of study and ensure that the schools' curriculum related to the attainment targets in each subject area. Primary schools are no longer in a position where they can block out the periods of time when students are on school practice and permit them to devise a curriculum which they would like to teach and which is, say, informed by a particular approach to primary education. The range of their replies is illustrated by the following:

It is a partnership. I would feed her [the student] ideas and suggestions related to the topic which had to be imposed because it is an integral part of the school's two-year plan. But wherever she has a strength or wishes to try something out I would be happy for her to have a try. ... I would prefer a student to keep to routines already established – basically this is for the children's sake. ... But she is free to try out and evaluate any different routines.

With the National Curriculum ... students must fit in with the school but within this the student should feel free to choose which aspects of a topic they wish to cover. ... I feel that teaching practice should be a time for students to experiment and try out different classroom practices, under the guidance of the mentor.

It [what is taught] is the school's responsibility, therefore it has to fit in with what has gone before and what comes after, so that the children get continuity. This is particularly so since the introduction of the National Curriculum. ... I feel because no two people would teach in the same way, a good deal has to be left to the student's choice. I oversee ... but how she sets about it is up to her.

Because this is the assessment term for Year 2 the school must determine largely what is taught. The student must fit in with school plans and relevant attainment targets. [With reference to how to teach] the mentor gives guidance because of her special knowledge of school resources. Otherwise great flexibility.

Summary

The body of evidence acquired from mentors, tutors and students is consistent and describes the circumstances which many primary students encounter during their periods of teaching practice. The National Curriculum with its programmes of study and attainment targets now shapes the primary school curriculum. The primary curriculum is so overloaded that virtually all schools have an overall school curriculum policy or plan which each teacher must follow reasonably closely. It is, therefore, understandable that the mentor teachers decided for students the areas of the curriculum that they had to cover or offered them some choice within prescribed limits. Within these constraints most mentors were prepared to discuss with students exactly what they would teach, especially where the curriculum allowed scope for flexibility. The subject area where this was least likely to happen was mathematics where the majority of schools required students to follow closely a published scheme of work specifically geared to the requirements of the National Curriculum.

While *what* was taught was circumscribed, mentors were prepared to allow students more scope in *how* they taught, in terms of choosing their methods and approaches to teaching. This is an area in which there was some inconsistency in the information. Students and their mentors reported that usually students were given some scope to decide how to teach while many tutors feel that students did not have that much flexibility in terms of deciding how they should teach. A possible explanation for this is that tutors have a broader appreciation than students and serving teachers of the variety of approaches to teaching, even when primary education is constrained and prescribed by the National Curriculum. They visit many different schools and experience the different ways in which the National Curriculum may be delivered, while students certainly, and mentors to some degree, are unlikely to have similarly wide-ranging experiences of alternative primary practices and teaching methods.

In the typical case, therefore, primary students on teaching practice can be regarded as being faced with a concrete and particular set of circumstances presented by the school in which they are, within limits, expected to teach a given curriculum. Students are placed in practical situations where they are usually required or expected to teach a given body of content in different subject or topic areas, although they are often offered some flexibility within parameters set by the National Curriculum. They are given greater scope in deciding for themselves the methods and approaches to adopt in their teaching. How, then, do they respond to this challenge and what resources do they call upon when preparing to teach and during their actual teaching?

Influences upon Students' Practical Teaching

The research entailed investigating the actual resources and information which students drew upon in their practical teaching and, particularly, for the purposes of this project, exploring how the contributions from their tutors and mentors informed and shaped their classroom practice. In order to consider these themes information was collected from two sources: (a) questions included in one of the interviews with the students which reviewed their practice and (b) the direct observation of their teaching in their practice classrooms followed immediately by a discussion about the lesson.

The interviews

Students were asked what advice and information has been particularly useful during their planning and day-to-day classroom practice. The aim was not to identify the actual information but its source, such as who had provided it. By this means it was intended to acquire evidence about the resources which students were drawing upon and which they had found particularly useful. The frequency with which different sources were mentioned is recorded in Table 8.1.

Source	Frequency
School-based	
Mentors	11
Other teachers	2
Training course based	
Practice tutors	9
Method tutors	4
Course work assignments	1
Social networks	
Friends and relatives	10
Other students	4
Books and journals	
Bright Ideas/Junior Education/Child Education	6
Others	3
Miscellaneous	
Previous school experience	2
Resource centre	1

Table 8.1 *Students' nominations of useful sources of information for planning teaching*

The evidence has to be regarded with some caution. Much of the information and advice which student teachers make use of in their practical teaching probably becomes 'absorbed' by them and taken on board or accepted as part of their working knowledge which, at a later time, they no longer specifically identify as being provided by a nominated source. For example, on a number of occasions the investigators noted that students were employing teaching suggestions which they knew were included in university-based curriculum method courses but during conversation the students did not refer to their method tutors as a particularly useful source. Nevertheless, the evidence is interesting and informative.

First it suggests that, broadly speaking, both mentors and tutors may be regarded as equally important sources for providing students with useful advice during their practical teaching. But there is another seemingly equally important group which students draw upon but which is never mentioned in the formal literature or discussions on teacher training, namely members of their social networks. Students are as equally likely to turn to other students or friends and relatives for advice. While training to be teachers students are not only involved in their training programme, be it school-based or university-based, they are also continuing to live and work within their communities and social environments. While it is difficult to assess the influence which members of social networks have upon students' preparation for practice they are clearly seen by students as a salient resource. These include other students, who pass on ideas which they have found to 'work' in their own teaching, and friends. Many of the friends and relatives mentioned were teachers, ranging from a close friend to 'boy friend's mother who is a teacher'.

Second it is instructive to note the publications which students say they found particularly useful. When answering the question the students were given no prompting but the majority mentioned very practically-oriented materials which provided them with suggestions for children's activities such as the *Bright Ideas* series, *Junior Education* and *Child Education*.

Direct observation of teaching

It is one thing to talk to student teachers about their teaching but to move beyond conjecture it is necessary to observe directly students' performances in the classroom so as to assess how tutors and mentors were influencing their actual teaching. In order to impose some rigour and structure upon the observations a particular procedure was devised.

Students were observed teaching for a complete lesson. During the lesson the observer identified a few key pedagogic incidents, usually two. These were instances when the student was actually engaged in intentional teaching activities and seeking to communicate lesson content to pupils or fostering their learning in some way. Incidents could include, for example: teacher-centred chalkboard expositions; organizing children working in groups using work cards; selecting and using artefacts for a science lesson; or developing a strategy to cope with an individual pupil's learning difficulties. Directly following the lesson the observer interviewed the student and engaged in conversation about the lesson with specific reference to the nominated pedagogic critical incidents. The purpose of the conversations was to try to establish what factors, considerations or advice had had some influence upon the student's pedagogical decision making before and during the lesson. When selecting pedagogical incidents there was no attempt to make a judgement about the quality of the student's teaching and during the interviews no reference was made to the quality of the student's teaching.

The observers made written notes during their observations and conversations and prepared a fair copy afterwards. The transcripts were scrutinized so as to identify the instances when students mentioned influences which had a bearing upon their pedagogical practices. These were then encoded within a category system derived from the data. No judgement was made about the quality of the influence or advice; even if it could be regarded as poor practice, it was still regarded as an influence. The categories which were generated from the data were as follows:

Student Influence

Grouped within this category are those instances where students made a specific effort to find out for themselves or in some way take the initiative when preparing material such as:

> I decided not to use a banda sheet because I wanted flexibility, allowing me to direct questions to individuals at the appropriate time in order to extend their grasp of probability.

> My own invention. Rather than producing another history worksheet (two already done this week) I thought that the children could get over what life on board ship was like through a letter home.

Common Sense

It was difficult to nominate an appropriate term, but 'common sense' seemed as satisfactory as any to embrace students' explanations for their pedagogical practices which refer to what may be termed their spontaneous dispositions to teach, where they use expressions such as common sense, obviousness or naturally, for example:

> My own common sense led me to choose things available at home plus something seen in school.

> ...because it seemed the simplest way of explaining effectively.

Class context and constraints

Students offered explanations for their classroom practices which related to their ongoing experiences with the class or constraints and circumstances inherent within their classrooms, such as:

> I realized [from] the ones used last week that I needed to redo them, making significant adjustments, as (a) the children had not grasped the notions involved; (b) too much was covered by one sheet; a simpler, briefer sheet was needed.

> I consider it to be an excellent source [referring to the atlas available in the class-room], very useful variety of appropriate representations of data. It was easily available and it seems sensible to use one source for the purposes of this lesson.

Mentors' influences

The mentor is mentioned by students as having some specific influence upon their teaching, for example:

> Decimal point 'diagram' came from a previous explanation given by the teacher.

> Did not give different sheets to different groups/individuals to match their ability levels as this was not the teacher's practice in this area.

Tutors' influences

A tutor (and it was usually a curriculum method tutor rather than the school practice supervisor) was mentioned by students as having had an influence upon their teaching, for example:

> The sentence label strips came from a tutor.

> The tutor gave valuable ideas and advice about the extension of a lesson he saw.

Other people's influences

From time to time students nominated other people besides teachers and tutors as having influenced their pedagogic practices, such as other students, relatives or friends, for instance:

> ...husband has an advertising studio and does posters frequently.

> I heard of the device through another student.

The number of times particular influences were mentioned are shown in Table 8.2.

Influence	Frequency
Student	53
Common sense	32
Context	31
Mentor	39
Tutor	41
Other person	28

Table 8.2 *Critical incidents; number of primary students' references to influences upon their teaching*

These data should be interpreted with caution and excessive reliance cannot be placed upon the frequency counts and variations between groups because, as mentioned at the outset, the information is, to a significant degree, shaped by the individual circumstances of school practice placements. The evidence indicates that students nominate tutors and mentors on roughly similar numbers of occasions as influencing their specific teaching acts. On a lesser number of occasions they mention other people. They are most likely to nominate themselves as the source which influenced their teaching, or the other factor which is closely associated with themselves namely that teaching is 'natural' or 'common sense'. Finally, the reason why they taught as they did could, to some degree, be attributed to contextual factors associated with their particular placement.

Discussion

There are a number of ways in which the information described in this chapter may be interpreted and incorporated into discussions about how students learn to become teachers and how they ought to be trained.

On the one hand, it may be argued (as it is by critics of university-based teacher education) that the evidence demonstrates that, from the point of view of student teachers as learners, teaching is very much a practical activity and that the only way in which to learn how to do it is through actual experience. Knowledge about teaching is 'situated knowledge' which is inextricably located within the physical and social context of its acquisition. Students devise strategies for making sense of the practical situations they find in particular classrooms so as to sustain ongoing events and resolve emergent problems and dilemmas. Students draw upon the obvious resources readily to hand, first of all themselves and their 'natural' and 'common sense' dispositions to teach and then help from their mentors and tutors. In addition, students live in a network of social relationships and they are also likely to refer to friends and relatives as a resource when planning their teaching. An evident implication which may easily be drawn is that since teaching is fundamentally a practical activity which relies upon common sense and the capability to cope with given circumstances, mentors and tutors may be regarded as useful in so far as they are able to help students to adapt successfully to the requirements and exigencies of the classrooms in which they learn to teach. This interpretation is informative in so far as it reminds us that, to some degree, becoming a teacher depends upon personal resources and dispositions and that the student teacher has to come to terms with and operate within a particular set of practical circumstances.

To envisage that solutions to any of teacher training's presumed ills or limitations can be remedied through policies which do little more than change the balance between the contributions of tutors and mentors is, in the light of this evidence, misguided. Teacher trainers who are not prepared to acknowledge the force of this characteristic of teacher training do themselves no service because whatever their aspirations and the content of their courses, actual circumstances have a potent effect upon how students learn to teach. But a whole-hearted acceptance of such a position reduces professional training to the unreflective reproduction of established practice, and even good practices should not be taken up without consideration.

On the other hand, it may be argued that while teacher training should be rooted in practice it must also extend and transcend notions of current good practice and those practices students encounter in particular schools. Student teachers may well (but should not) 'work it out for themselves' or call upon the support of relatives and friends, but what is crucial in terms of developing professional capability is the quality and suitability of the advice and support that students receive and their capacity to reflect upon it and incorporate it in their own teaching. For a student teacher to use a teaching tactic on the grounds that their friend used it in their school or to engage in a teaching act because it is 'common sense' (which probably means that it is what they experienced in their own schooling) does little more than reproduce well-worn teaching routines; it hardly counts as informed professional practice. In particular it encourages an approach which regards teaching as 'doing things' with children. The teacher's task (even within the aspirations and constraints of the National Curriculum) becomes one of providing activities for children and making use of other people and their experience and expertise for suggestions and advice about what to 'do'. What, of course, is neglected is the focus upon children's learning and providing the appropriate learning tasks and activities which are related to different pupils' abilities and which are intended to advance learning. Advice from relatives or magazines about lesson content or activities counts for little unless it can be related to the prior learning experiences and abilities of the children in a particular class. It is one thing to call upon convenient sources when planning practical teaching but it must be stressed that the quality of the forthcoming teaching will depend crucially upon the quality of the information and help proffered. It is in this respect that the contributions of the mentor and tutor are important and what matters is the quality of the advice that they provide which should have regard for the effective promotion of learning in a specific class of children with their various abilities and aptitudes.

The limitation of this research and, indeed, the limitation of most research in the field is the failure to address the issue of the quality of the information and advice provided for student teachers. This is understandable since the methodological and conceptual problems entailed when investigating this issue are daunting. One theme which is embedded in the interview evidence, but which it is very difficult to quantify, is the concern with quality. Since it was not built into the research, only some speculative comments about 'quality' may be made. Students often volunteered the observation that the source of the advice and information they received was not all that important, what mattered was the quality and utility of the information provided and whether it was given in a helpful and supportive manner. Whether it was a tutor or a mentor was of little consequence to the student.

To some degree, teaching skill is a capability which beginners must acquire and develop for themselves. But it is precisely because the uninformed may regard teaching as a job which any graduate with subject knowledge or mature person with experience of life can pick up by 'being thrown in at the deep end' that the dangers of sitting next to Nellie or Nigel must be guarded against. There is a clear implication for school-based models of teacher training which emphasize the role of mentors. The effective mentor has a special contribution to make in developing the student's teaching. The mentor should have a sensitive appreciation of the children's prior learning and abilities so that he or she is uniquely placed to offer that particular advice about the circumstances of his or her class and the children within it which the student should bear in mind when planning to support and foster learning. This, of course, is appreciated by many mentors.

Summary

Student teachers are placed in training contexts where they will, necessarily, regard teaching as essentially a practical activity; one in which they must respond to ongoing events and promote learning in concrete and particular circumstances. A major priority for mentors should be to draw upon their expertise and knowledge of particular classes so as to provide students with the help and advice which supports their effectiveness as teachers within the special conditions and constraints they find in their practice classrooms.

In addition, teacher training should be concerned with all-round professional development and the beginner should acquire a wider appreciation of his or her role and become familiar with alternative approaches to primary practice and be aware of their strengths and possible limitations. Students must also gain some idea of how good or effective their own performance is when compared with that of other students and, most importantly, they need to know whether the particular circumstances of their class and school may have hindered or fostered their professional development. It is, of course, possible for context-specific knowledge acquired in one situation to be developed and applied in other circumstances but this necessary dimension to professional training needs to be specially encouraged. It is precisely because tutors are removed from the day-to-day life of classrooms that they are strategically placed to foster this essential dimension of teacher education.

Neither tutors nor mentors are more important parties to initial teacher training; both make equally worthwhile, but different, contributions.

Notes

* For full details of the review of relevant literature and the research design see David McNamara (1993), *Student Teachers' Classroom Practice: The influence of their tutors and mentors*, The University of Hull.

The research reported in this chapter was supported by the Paul Hamlyn Foundation.

Chapter 9

The Role of the Mentor in Secondary Schools

Judith Dormer

Introduction

This chapter examines the role of the mentor in secondary schools at a time when both schools and higher education institutions (HEIs) are seeking to rethink their changing roles and responsibilities. With the onset of radical changes in the nature of initial teacher education (ITE) and the growing awareness of the need for a longitudinal approach to induction and staff development, the appointment of mentors in schools has become commonplace. The term 'mentor' is used to describe the differing roles of supervisory teachers in a variety of school-based schemes for ITE, including both articled and licensed teacher schemes. Mentors are used in the induction of teachers at many stages in their careers. In particular the transfer of training into schools announced by Kenneth Clarke in 1992 has meant increasing responsibility for mentors. The rapid nature of these changes has meant that teachers have been thrust into the role of mentor, while uncertainty still exists about the fundamental nature of the task they are to perform.

Definitions vary from Wilkin's (1992) interpretation of a mentor as teacher trainer, to Crossland's (1991) notion of 'critical friend'. As a practising teacher at the sharp end of these innovations, not only have I been aware of local initiatives in mentor training, but I have become personally involved in two mentoring schemes. First, with neither training nor clear guidelines, I mentored an Articled Teacher during the final year of his two-year course and as a result felt that whilst supporting him adequately, I had not managed to provide the structured framework which would have encouraged his professional development more fully. Second, I was asked to become a subject mentor in a pilot school-based scheme for training postgraduate (PGCE) students. Partly as a result of reflection upon my earlier mentoring practice (and in anticipation of the second) I undertook a research project which studied recent experiences of mentoring in East Devon secondary schools.

Aims of the Research Project

My aims were twofold:

- to attempt to clarify the mentor's role as it is currently being interpreted
- to try to define a model of effective mentoring suitable for the continuum of teacher education from ITE to induction and staff development.

The intention was to examine mentoring practice and to attempt to ascertain the needs of mentors and their protégés (I use the term 'protégé' in preference to 'mentee'). If my own early experience was confirmed, and mentors had been left to generate their own roles, it might be helpful to provide them with a framework for conceptualizing their roles and to assist them in improving their practice.

The research process

Data collection took place in three phases, during the period from Spring to Autumn 1993.

Phase 1
In order to provide data for the first of my aims – the attempted clarification of the mentor's role as it is currently being conceptualized and practised – questionnaires were sent to the 15 secondary schools in the East Devon area. In these questionnaires respondents were asked for their definition of:

- the term 'mentor'
- the main functions of a mentor
- the most important qualities a mentor should possess.

I hoped that the responses to these questionnaires would provide schools who were willing to participate in the second phase of research and would suggest suitable topics for discussion in interviews.

Phase 2
The main phase of the data collection took the form of semi-structured interviews with personnel involved in many stages of the mentoring process:

deputy heads, subject mentors, newly qualified teachers (NQTs), returners to the profession and PGCE students in the final term of their training. Most of the personnel interviewed came from two of the schools in the original sample. These schools were selected using the following criteria:

- they were both willing, and in fact keen, to take part in the study
- they had a wide range of experience of mentoring both in ITE and in staff development and support
- the views of staff would be sampled from a very large school (over 2000 pupils) and one that was comparatively small (500 to 1000 pupils)
- opinions of colleagues who were preparing, as I was, to take part in the pilot PGCE scheme would be examined, as well as the perceptions of those who were not involved in such a scheme.

A total of 18 personnel were interviewed, including seven mentor pairs.

Phase 3
Phase 3 used questionnaires to explore the progress of some of the PGCE students as they took up posts as NQTs the following Autumn. Whereas phase 2 involved a snapshot of a range of colleagues, the aim of phase 3 was to discover the reactions of the same students to the mentoring process at a different point in their careers.

Results of the investigation

Phase 1 responses
Completed questionnaires were returned by 11 of the 15 schools (73 per cent). The views expressed were those of the person in overall charge of staff development and fell into three broad categories which emphasized:

- the *support* given by the mentor
- the *professional development* of the protégé
- the *empowering* or *managerial* role of the mentor.

Responses which fell mainly into the first category included:

understanding, patience, encouragement, trust, empathy, friendship, counselling/listening skills, mediation, liaise, look after interests, appreciation of problems, advice, support, guidance, common sense, sense of proportion.

Those in the broadly developmental area included:

resource professional development, challenge, criticize constructively, critical friend, help to develop your own answers, smooth transition, organize, teach, teacher trainer, specialist educator, professional tutor.

Those in the third area seemed to suggest notions of oversight, the overview, enabler in general, inferring that someone experienced in the school structure/hierarchy is needed:

authority, experience, knowledge, vision, clear idea of goals, ability to do the job, efficient senior colleague, see job in context, appraise, institutional loyalty.

As might be expected from the responses of colleagues already in a managerial capacity, the support and professional development of the individual are considered, but this is underpinned by an awareness of whole-school structure and needs.

Phase 2 responses: the data collected from semi-structured interviews
As a mentor, I was aware that mentoring tends to be subjective in its judgements and personal to the individuals concerned. Although in the future its use as a method of training may require a more formalized structure, it was my belief at this stage in my research that its success or failure depends on the commitment of the mentor and the quality of the relationships developed between mentor and protégé. Therefore I decided that the use of semi-structured interviews incorporating open-ended questions was the most appropriate method to gather rich anecdotal material suitable for qualitative analysis.

Having already identified both institutions and personnel from whom I wished to gather data, interview schedules were devised. The questions addressed themes arising from both the questionnaires used in phase 1 and from the relevant literature. Both the format and number of questions were adapted to suit the professional status of the person being interviewed. All respondents were asked to comment on the role, functions of and qualities desirable in a mentor. They were also asked to comment on their own experience, with particular reference to the support they were given, the time spent in association with the mentor, or protégé, and the availability of the mentor. All respondents were asked to comment on the nature of the assessment in which they were engaged and whether it conflicted with the mentor's supportive role. As the use of tape-recorders can be inhibiting, responses were recorded on pre-prepared forms, and all respondents were given the opportunity to check the accuracy of the material.

THE VIEWS OF PGCE STUDENTS

The comments of the PGCE students fell broadly into the two main categories of support and challenge with overtones of the managerial/empowering aspect more muted than in the original survey. Interpersonal skills of counselling, listening 'and to hear what's going on underneath', patience, humour, empathy, inspiration, motivation, commitment, approachability and encouragement were among the qualities mentioned under the umbrella of 'support', as were the need for guidance and resourcing for specific skills. Knowing what to provide and *when* to provide it was felt to be essential. The area of resourcing and developing skills appears to be the link between support and challenge. Once more there is a delicate balance: '*supportive* rather than intrusive – that's a difficult divide – not too structured – give you autonomy but also good advice when needed'. They wanted practical help with classroom management and lesson preparation 'the nuts and bolts of teaching' from someone with a 'broad base of skills'.

The theme of challenge to inspire real progress and development was taken up when exploring whether the role of assessor conflicts with that of the mentor as supporter. They were unanimous in feeling that the school-based mentor should not only be part of the assessment process (as indeed they already are), but that if professionally done, and with a good mentor/protégé relationship, it was a crucial part of the student's development: 'Ongoing assessment was constructive and developmental...wasn't threatening. ...Criticism and challenge is needed to help you develop'. One student came up with his own equivalent of the 'critical friend'. 'If they're professional they should be capable of objective involvement.' Students seemed to have no doubt that mentors were capable of achieving this apparent paradox!

Most students felt that they had adequate support from school-based mentors, most of whom were subject-based. They found their mentors very accessible, although mostly in an informal way, as there was no formally allotted meeting time. The need for a degree of challenge was indicated in the desire for a greater degree of observation and feedback: 'Accessible... adequate support. I would have liked more observation and feedback ongoing through the practice'.

The notion of the mentor as a figure of authority in the hierarchical structure of the school did not figure greatly, except in more general terms: 'elder, wiser, experienced, oversees, refers...'.

THE VIEWS OF NQTS

It was only possible to interview two NQTs at this stage. With such a small number any conclusions drawn must be tentative. However the mentors of both NQTs were also interviewed, thereby giving a more rounded picture.

Both NQTs had nearly completed their first year's teaching and expressed initial confusion as to who their appointed mentor was, and identified the need for early support: 'sympathy — they should remember what it's like to be new, not only to teaching but to the school...be more proactive...nip things in the bud...'.

Questions about the degree of assessment elicited the following response:

> There was no open assessment that I was aware of and certainly none discussed. The deputy head i/c personnel came in my lesson once but not in the position of mentor and there was no detailed feedback.

The need for development and formative assessment was strongly signalled by one NQT and a new aspect of the mentoring role began to emerge:

> ...someone to give career direction...a position of power in the school...someone to respect... . Listening but follows listening with action. Very accessible socially but no formally prescribed time...no checking or evaluation of lessons...I feel very strongly that more formal support is both needed and desirable.

The other NQT reflected on the nature of assessment: 'My mentor will be my appraiser. She has assessed my teaching and made comments. The roles are not conflicting — it's vital to A-level development'.

It seems that in their references to career development and appraisal, both NQTs are flagging the difference between mentoring students and mentoring NQTs. Their differing needs require a change in style by the mentor. Both groups have shown the need for observation, feedback and hence development, but these NQTs are asking more strongly for structured support and are aware of the role of assessment and appraisal in career development. As students approach NQT status good mentoring practice will need to acknowledge these requirements.

THE VIEWS OF RETURNERS TO THE PROFESSION

The two returners interviewed stressed the need for mentors to fulfil a supportive role. Both moral and practical guidance were needed and they wanted to be given confidence, reassurance and help in updating their skills and knowledge of subject matter: 'Basic things about school layout — how to behave...lent me books. Very helpful to have someone...so as not to be wasting people's time.'

The only element of challenge came when mentioning the need for feedback and when discussing the role of the mentor as assessor. Here for the first time there was an awareness that the need for assessment could be inhibiting:

> A critical friend – appraisal rather than assessment as part of the supportive role. There was no formal assessment which could have been conflicting – although material for a reference arose because of her involvement in mentoring.

THE VIEWS OF SUBJECT MENTORS

Subject mentors' comments once more fell into the categories of support (both moral and practical) and challenge (in the sense of encouraging development) but with a clearer sense of the institutional structure. Empathy, rapport, the ability to inspire and motivate, were all stressed as necessary, together with the need to provide practical help, ideas and coping strategies at the classroom level. One mentor was emphatic that she was not an expert or a role model, but working alongside the protégé, and coordinating experiences. Subject mentors saw themselves as 'a sounding board...the first port of call' but were also very aware of the importance of three major issues. First, the necessity of acting as enabler or possible bridge with senior management:

> ...negotiator, giving practical and career advice, someone with enough authority or experience to suggest possible routes, the ability to see things in perspective...to take an overview...

Second, the importance of the crucial balance between support and challenge became apparent as they discussed *when* and *how* to step in. It was felt that there was a danger of allowing negativity to develop if help was only reactive. Students should be 'helped to find limits about what they can realistically hope to achieve' but that they should still be:

> encouraged to be brave enough to try out ideas if theirs don't always work...helped to develop their own ideas – develop self-criticism...gradually encouraging her to take more responsibility for getting the feel of standards which are sometimes nebulous...believe in her judgements.

They felt strongly that as mentors they should be aware and proactive and 'give the fruits of knowledge and experience – even when unsolicited...Pursue problem areas'.

Third, whilst feeling that there must be a clear structure within the school and especially more time to do the job properly, ('I'm not sure I'm paid enough for the time and commitment!') the need for careful pairing and adaptability by the mentor to that particular protégé's needs was stressed: 'It would be destructive to impose a prescriptive model....I respond to need...it goes back to what I said about empathy...there must be a suitable pairing...'.

The theme of a suitable pairing was felt to be important if the mentor were to act as assessor, with a mechanism built in for withdrawal if the relationship did not work. However, five out of the seven mentors stated clearly that assessment was a positive part of the mentoring role and should be 'open, sensitive direction...in their best interests giving career advice where necessary...criticism should be a challenge to further development!'

Two mentors replied that they had a responsibility to the school, the profession and the pupils, to weed out unsuitable candidates and that this was also in the students' best interests. One mentor felt that it would conflict by changing the relationship:

> It must be made clear...'I'm not assessing you!' – it would undermine the relationship...should be supportively critical but not judgemental...wouldn't be able to admit weaknesses.

All the mentors felt they were accessible, but that time was a problem and should be available formally. One mentor admitted to feeling very 'hassled' at times, giving up time both in the lunch hour and after school.

THE VIEWS OF CO-TUTORS

The term 'co-tutor' is used for the person with overall responsibility for personnel/mentoring in school-based ITE. It is adopted from the pilot scheme currently being developed by St Luke's School of Education, University of Exeter. The comments of the co-tutors, although advocating support, encouragement, patience and guidance (as might be expected) emphasized the more developmental skills:

> experience, communication skills – both listening and interviewing; counselling skills – supporting someone in their development of decision making; providing inset opportunities; regular consultation.

Both co-tutors felt strongly that assessment *was* part of the mentor's role, was *not* conflicting and was both necessary and desirable for satisfactory development:

> It's no different from a teacher assessing a pupil! There's nothing threatening about the assessment process for anybody – it's part of the educative process. You can't be supportive without being positively critical....Part of the mentor's skill is involving the student in negotiation during the assessment process.

Phase 3 responses

Three out of the original five PGCE students returned completed question-naires. Two had completed their first half-term as NQTs, whilst the third had not yet obtained a teaching post. The somewhat limited data collected support the notion that, even during the short time span of this research, sys-tems for mentoring are already becoming more formalized. In both their respective schools the NQTs were aware of their mentor from the start and formal induction programmes were in operation. It was felt that there was continuity with earlier training, and that the progression from student to NQT was recognized:

> The induction meetings often address issues which were an integral part of the PGCE for example, class management...I don't feel that I have been cush-ioned as such, therefore providing the necessary challenge, but I know that support is readily available.

The Emergence of an Alternative Model

It was at this point, after constantly rereading and reacting with the data and the opinions and personalities of the respondents that I returned to the literature on mentoring. Earlier in my research, whilst reflecting on my own mentoring practice, I had found Daloz's (1986) model of challenge and sup-port (see Figure 9.1) particularly helpful. It was developed while he was mentoring adult learners in the United States and seemed to support my view of my own experience and the views of many of my respondents that a combination of high support and high challenge are necessary for optimum professional development. Daloz also sees a third element to be necessary to the successful mentoring practice – vision.

My understanding of his theoretical framework for use in adult education and my own 'hands-on' experience of colleagues and their needs were com-bined to propose a model which might be suitable for today's changing envi-ronment of school-based ITE, continuing staff development and appraisal. This model contains the three dimensions of support, challenge and vision identified by Daloz, which were apparent in the research data. However it operates on two levels, each appropriate to the differing experience and needs of the protégé and the position of the mentor in the organization (see Figure 9.2).

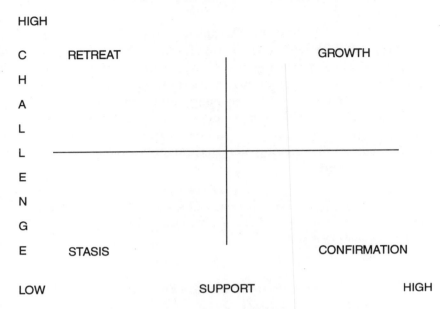

Figure 9.1 *Daloz's model of challenge and support*

Although I see level 1 as applying primarily to students and level 2 to NQTs and further professional development, this will not always be the case. It will depend both on the stage of the protégé in their career development, (they may need level 1-type support *immediately after* promotion or appointment) and on the position of the mentor in the establishment.

This model however does not demonstrate Daloz's conclusions on the effect of high/low challenge/support on the protégé. An alternative model is proposed therefore (see Figure 9.3) which is applicable to staff development and is based primarily on my observations of the progress of the NQTs interviewed in phase 2. The NQT who had experienced a high level of support and structured development and who did have a clear understanding of the mentor's role in her progress, achieved early promotion!

I put forward this extension tentatively as a positive model for future examination. Within the data collected I have seen some evidence for the quadrants relating to high challenge/high support and low challenge/high support but the other sections are a result of my own reflection on observation of colleagues over the years.

DIMENSION 1: SUPPORT

STUDENTS (LEVEL 1)
Empathy; building confidence; listening; developing trust; provision of a 'holding' environment
NQTs (LEVEL 2)
Providing structure and a sense of identity and a place within it; enabling; the emergence of mutual benefit/sense of purpose

DIMENSION 2: CHALLENGE

STUDENTS (LEVEL 1)
Stimulation by provision of ideas/resources; diagnostic formative assessment by negotiation as a form of continuous development; positive expectations
NQTs (LEVEL 2)
Providing professional development/career opportunities; mainly summative assessment including possible appraisal/job references

DIMENSION 3: VISION

STUDENTS (LEVEL 1)
Inspiration and motivation; reflection on theory and practice
NQTs (LEVEL 2)
The overview of the institution; awareness of developing initiatives and current trends; wise placement in new appointments; wisdom in choice of mentor

Figure 9.2 *An extended two-level model of challenge, support and development*

Conclusion

The main conclusions arising from this study are that:

- the mentor can no longer be simply regarded as a 'critical friend'; the protégé needs a different relationship with the mentor according to his or her level of experience
- the returner will need a high level of support and confidence

HIGH CHALLENGE/LOW SUPPORT	HIGH CHALLENGE/HIGH SUPPORT
Attempts initiatives/career progress without reflecting on teaching/pupil needs.	Confident reflective practitioner progressing up the organization.
LOW CHALLENGE/LOW SUPPORT	LOW CHALLENGE/HIGH SUPPORT
Lacks confidence. Disillusioned with teaching/establishment.	Personal loyalty to colleagues and pupils. Remain entrenched in existing practices – little career progress.

Figure 9.3 *Model based on Elliot and Calderhead's extension of Daloz's model (Elliot and Calderhead, 1993)*

- the model of support/challenge/vision provides a framework to help mentors diagnose their protégés' needs, thus enabling both parties to proceed with confidence
- the nature of assessment should be overt and understood by both mentor and protégé; in this way it is less likely to be an area for possible conflict and more likely to become positive and developmental
- adequate resourcing in terms of training (especially time for mentors to carry out their role properly and professionally) is essential. Mentors need to feel their role is valued.

It is heartening to note that not only are more structured schemes coming into place to help define the mentor's role but that the School Teachers' Review Body in its annual report had as one of its key recommendations that headteachers should have a duty to provide adequate support for NQTs. The other side of the coin is that Harrow public school has recently withdrawn from school-based ITE because the increased workload to mentors is perceived as threatening the quality of their teaching (Pyke, 1994). The transfer of responsibility for ITE to schools inevitably means that school staff will need to develop new skills. As school-based ITE becomes more firmly established and mentors become skilled practitioners, it is to be hoped that the value of their contribution will be recognized and adequately resourced.

References

Crossland, H (1991) 'A competency-based approach to teacher development at the induction phase', unpublished course notes, University of Plymouth.

Daloz, L A (1986) *Effective Teaching and Mentoring*, San Francisco, CA: Jossey-Bass.

Elliot, B and Calderhead, J (1993) 'Mentoring for teacher development: possibilities and caveats', in McIntyre, D, Hagger, H and Wilkin, M (eds) *Mentoring: Perspectives on School-Based Teacher Education*, London: Kogan Page.

Pyke, N (1994) 'Harrow hasn't the time for trainees', *The Times Educational Supplement*, p.3, 11/2/94.

Wilkin, M (ed) (1992) *Mentoring in Schools*, London: Kogan Page.

Chapter 10

Supervision Strategies and their Application in the School Context

Anne Proctor

Introduction

In the rush to locate teacher training in school and to give teachers the responsibility for that training, it would be a pity if all the exploratory work already undertaken in this area of expertise is ignored or discounted. This must apply particularly to the work on tutors' supervision of the practical teaching component of teacher training. As the importance of the professional skill required in supervision has been recognized, so a body of research has been developed to explore its nature and potential. Presumably at least some of this work will have relevance in the development of mentor or teacher tutor training programmes. The danger is that it may not be taken seriously in some quarters because it is associated with the world of training institutions and hence a supposedly inappropriate approach to the development of trainee teachers' skills.

Much of the early work in the area of supervision of student teaching was concerned with defining the complementary roles of tutors from the training institutions and the cooperating teachers working with students in classrooms. On the one hand tutors were described as being out of touch with the classroom situation and superfluous to the enterprise whereas teachers offered practical, realistic help and cooperated with student teachers to minimize the influence of the tutor. On the other hand it was suggested that tutors had an important role in developing effective professional relationships, in supporting the student teachers and ensuring a quality experience for them whereas, it was suggested, teachers often neglected to help students with basic classroom skills, were unaware of how they themselves functioned in their classrooms and lacked the wider vision to help student teachers generalize from their experiences. There has been much more agreement however about the very real difficulties faced by trios (student teachers, teachers and tutors) trying to work together without putting the student teachers under the impossible strain of trying to please both teachers and tutors who were in disagreement.

Grimmett and Ratzloff (1986) suggested that at the time of writing 'clear and differentiated supervision roles are conspicuously absent, leading in some cases to duplication of function, in others to omission'. However, not all the studies have been so pessimistic. For example, Stones (1984) has described how teachers, students and tutors can cooperate by using a common model for professional development, and programmes such as the Oxford Internship Scheme show the effective cooperation and definition of roles which comes from careful consultation.

Some studies have focused on how tutors work with student teachers, the factors to which they give attention and how the emphasis in supervision changes as student teachers become more proficient. It is interesting to learn that tutors want to be seen as teachers by the students; that their practice is often less effective as they try to identify with teachers; that they themselves get better with experience (Rust, 1988) and that they adapt their practice to fit the situation in which they are placed (Proctor, 1993). Like many other people, tutors do not always do what they say they do or what they say they believe in.

There is no reason to believe that teachers in their role as trainers of student teachers in school will not also be influenced by particular factors in the classrooms in which they work. It is quite likely that sometimes they also will fail to act in a totally consistent way and it may be very helpful for them to explore some of the actions which tutors have taken, if only to understand better the influences which they themselves may feel in their new mentoring role.

The purpose of this chapter is to consider ways in which tutors apply their knowledge about supervision in particular contexts. Although supervision as suggested above is often described as a very inexact skill, more recent work has shown how tutors adapt their strategies to meet the needs of the student teachers they supervise (Proctor, 1991). It is this information which may be of value to teachers in their new role as mentors.

After distinguishing between the complementary roles of professional supervision of student teachers and counselling, this chapter considers some strategies for supervision, illustrated by examples taken from case-study material. The way tutors make decisions about when to use any particular approach and the factors in a situation which will influence those decisions are then explored.

Supervision and Counselling

Much of the recent work on mentoring gives the impression that supervision and counselling are synonymous. Clearly the roles of supervision and counselling are complementary but it is helpful to make some distinctions:

Supervision is considered to be particularly concerned with aspects of:

- observing and analysing teaching/learning situations
- identifying and helping others to identify pertinent aspects of teaching in different situations
- using strategies to help others to achieve identified professional goals
- assessing, evaluating and recording, cooperatively, professional development of self and others.

Related to the role of supervision, counselling is particularly concerned with aspects of:

- sensitivity to and perception of the needs of a mentor
- skills in helping people to express themselves and their feelings and to understand their own needs so that they are better able to draw on their own resources in meeting those needs.

The subsequent discussion is focused primarily on aspects of supervision as defined above since much of the work on mentoring seems to neglect this aspect. In that the two cannot be totally separated in practice, the complementary role of counselling will be referred to at appropriate times.

Supervision Strategies

Instruction in professional skills

Teachers and tutors alike will recognize the importance of offering instruction to student teachers. This may take a number of forms and apply to many different aspects of classroom practice. For example teachers may:

- show how to put up a display
- explain the need for children to line up at particular times
- model the introduction to a teaching session
- help to prepare a class for a practical activity while explaining how it is done
- show by instruction and example how to develop questioning techniques.

Sometimes instruction can come in the form of 'first aid' to a new student teacher, eg, 'Don't let the 5-year olds all go out for paint at the same time'. It may/should include justification for the advice.

Many, perhaps most, professional skills are complex, made up of simpler skills. At the same time professionals are required to make careful judgements about how and when to apply the skill or adapt it to a particular situation. However, this does not negate the value of instruction but only influences the way the directions are presented by a supervising tutor or teacher. If skill teaching is to be successful it requires that the skill is broken down into component parts, that the learner is able to practise the parts, put them together and receive feedback on the performance. Most importantly the learner needs to begin to understand when the skill is appropriate and how to adapt it to the given situation. It is these elements of critical analysis and subsequent modification which make teaching a *professional* skill. In other words a professional skill has the following characteristics:

- competence in performing the elements of the skill
- ability to assess the context in which the skill will be applied, by recognizing similarities and differences with previous experiences
- adapting a known skill or amalgamating elements of known skills to meet the needs of the new situation.

Some extracts from tutors' notes to student teachers show the attempts of the tutors to offer help in the analysis of a context and development of specific skills. (The extracts are only part of the comments given to the student teachers.)

Tutor A/student 1 (year 6)

> Your instructions were clear and unhurried and you held out for the level of attention that you required from the children. The latter were involved from the outset by your skilful use of the questions, and settled down to their tasks remarkably quickly. I must own up to being pleasantly surprised by the standard of their folder covers. I thought that they might have required more detailed instructions about lettering and layout than you actually gave them – but the end product would seem to indicate that this was not the case. However, in future lessons like this I think you will find that it pays rich dividends if you pay attention to the following points:
>
> (i) Get the children to set out a border – it keeps the work neat and leaves a margin for error
> (ii) Give detailed instructions regarding the size and type of lettering that you require. Possibly even specify a layout for the work
> (iii) Perhaps specify figure/ground relationship between lettering and illustration.

In the notes the tutor establishes the context within which the student teacher is working and gives positive reinforcement to certain aspects of the teaching which were effective. By picking out some aspects of this classroom he gives the student teacher some cues to help in contextualizing in another situation. He then goes on to give very precise instructions about how he believed that activity would best be achieved. If he were then able to see the student teacher applying these skills at a later stage he would be in a position to give feedback.

Tutor B/student 2 (year 4)

1. When the children were reading out loud, you could have used some strategies to help the rest to keep attention, eg:

- don't give the quiet readers too long a time to read as their voices begin to tail off
- help the children to speak up and slowly in order that they may be heard
- sometimes recap on the story to make sure that nobody is lost.

And later, in the same set of notes:

It was the preparation for your writing session which rather surprised me. You seemed very uncertain about exactly what you wanted to do, with the result that you tried to achieve too much. I think that you wanted the children to relate the story as though they were reporting it and, in fact, put it in a newspaper format. If this is the case then you could have helped them to outline the contents, perhaps putting guidelines on the board. With that clear, you could then have very briefly outlined the format without going into the structure of a newspaper. The latter could not be achieved in the time you had available. In fact, when you returned to the children's writing your guidelines were fairly clear. I think that it would help you if we discuss some of your plans in detail in order to identify the really important elements.

In this instance these instructions are not quite so specific as those of tutor A because the discussion is about more complex issues than preparing a folder. However, they still give quite precise information picking out aspects of the context and some specific teaching skills. What was apparent to the tutor, and will also be apparent to the reader, was that the complexity of the ideas and their location in context would require a joint planning session between tutor and student. It would be in such a face-to face discussion that instructional support could be given and then followed through in the classroom.

Developing a professional dialogue

Instruction may be one effective way of sharing professional skills but certainly it is not a sufficient way. The way one teacher carries out an activity is different from the way in which another teacher does a similar activity. The decision about when a particular teaching approach may be appropriate is a matter for thoughtful judgement, not for unthinking application. In the first example above, the tutor offered careful help in the skill of giving instructions, but the question of whether it was necessary to give such precise instructions to the children in that particular context is a matter for critical analysis and reflection. A student teacher who is facing substantial difficulties in the classroom will need some quite systematic support in developing appropriate strategies, as in the case of the second example. However, as student teachers develop their professional competences, it is increasingly important that they reflect upon their choice of strategies and consider whether alternative ways would be even more effective. At the same time they will want to reconsider what they wish to achieve in their teaching and relate this to the chosen strategy or approach. The literature suggests that there are two main approaches to developing this thinking and reflective attitude.

One way is illustrated by the clinical approaches to supervision (Cogan, 1973). Under these circumstances the supervising tutor is a resource who contributes under the direction of the student teacher. It becomes the responsibility of the student teacher to decide to which particular professional focus she or he wishes to give attention. Having made that decision she or he then invites the tutor to make an identified contribution. An extract from tutor notes illustrates where this may be appropriate:

Tutor C/student 3 (year 2)

> Your high standards both in planning and evaluation continue. The high standard you set for yourself is transmitted to the children in many interesting ways. They arrive at school anticipating what is to come and during discussion they are eager to share ideas. They really do listen to each other's contribution. I have yet to see a bored face in this classroom. You are obviously matching activities to children's levels in all areas. The book contribution is going well and a most valuable learning experience recognizing that their writing is for an audience. Suggestions from last week have been acted on immediately. You have been sensitive to possible problems and the display is so interesting.

In this instance the tutor is making evaluative comments, all of a positive nature, reinforcing aspects of the teaching in which the student teacher is doing well. In this very positive context there is now room for a new emphasis to be chosen. In other words the tutor will want to consider what contribution she can make, at this stage, to the professional development of a student teacher who is being so successful. The clinical supervision approach offers an effective strategy by which the student teacher will identify those aspects of professional practice which have become important for him or her. This may be to identify why certain aspects are so successful or perhaps to confirm the 'match' between the work set for the children and their individual needs. The important point is that the responsibility will be the student teacher's with the tutor acting as a resource in responding to direct requests.

A second way of developing a thinking and reflective attitude is the psychopedagogical approach. This is also intended to stimulate dialogue in a situation where a student teacher is achieving at least a fair degree of success in the classroom. The approach contrasts with that above, in that the tutor takes the initiative by recommending a particular theoretical approach and applying that theory to the classroom situation. This can be illustrated in the work of Stones (1984) who advocates a psychopedagogical approach to supervision. He argues that to be effective teaching must be subject to scrutiny. If practice is ever to improve then it must draw on appropriate theoretical insights in a planned and determined way. He advocates a quite formal approach to ensuring that this happens. Student teachers along with mentors identify objectives for children's learning. In the light of insights from theory the appropriateness of the objectives will be assessed and a suitable way of achieving them will be agreed. As the teaching is implemented so it will be evaluated in terms of the outcomes and appropriate theoretical insights. The associated analysis will form the basis for professional dialogue. Stones' approach requires that teacher, student teacher and tutor are all aware of this particular procedure for planning and implementation and are prepared to follow it. However, the same ideas can be applied in a slightly less comprehensive way by the tutor sharing particular theoretical insights as part of the normal classroom observation and subsequent discussion and this is illustrated in the work of Cohn and Gellman (1988) in the USA as well as being typical of similar approaches in this country. The extracts below demonstrate the potential for this approach.

Tutor D/student 4 (year 6)

Also – energy is a very broad concept – you were introducing a great many concepts/ideas all at once. Even with the fact sheet available and a TV programme to come, you need some visual aid(s) to help the children to envisage, say, a solar panel, barrage in a river/lake, etc.

After talking to the children it became fairly clear that they really just did not know what energy was. Looking at your lesson plan, even with the help of the worksheet, children just wouldn't have understood.

The notes show that the tutor is dealing with some important factors to do with the way the children learn and the most appropriate matching teaching strategies. It would be quite easy to see this session being followed by a dialogue about principles of children's cognitive development and learning which could lead to some detailed planning based on those principles.

Implementing Supervision Strategies

Clearly the above strategies are not discrete or used quite independently of one another. A mentor/supervisor will know about and use a range of strategies.

In an extensive examination of tutors' actions as supervisors undertaken over a two-year period by the writer, it became quite clear that supervision strategies were used in response to the different situations in which tutors found themselves. Experienced tutors were responsive to the needs of the student teachers and the context of the block school experience. This meant that they took into account the competency of the student teacher, the degree and quality of the support provided by the teacher, the specific school requirements, the nature of the curriculum in that school and the characteristics of the class in which the student teacher was teaching. In making judgements about their actions tutors referred to:

- what the student was able to achieve
- the capability of the class teacher to contribute
- the general demands of the school and the specific demands of the class
- the personal relationships of the situation,

but it was the interaction of these together which influenced the tutors' actions. To summarize: the tutor acted on the basis of what she or he believed the student teacher could achieve in that situation. It was by an examination of these actions and the judgements which prompted them that supervision could become more effective.

This can be made clearer by taking the examples outlined above and trying to locate them in their contexts.

Tutor B/student 2

This example was given to illustrate an instructional approach to supervision. Of interest here is whether the context can tell us anything about why that strategy should be used and whether an alternative one would have been more appropriate.

Student 2 was undertaking a seven-week block school experience. Although he was working with an experienced and supportive teacher, she was not at that stage offering systematic help of an instructional nature. For a number of reasons student 2 was not achieving success. His preparation was conscientious but ineffective and he was rapidly losing the interest and cooperation of the class. Action by the teacher and the tutor was essential. The evidence from the study referred to above suggested that under these circumstances the most appropriate action was to offer a limited instructional approach. A student teacher who is no longer in touch with a class needs some clear advice about how to remedy the situation as quickly as possible, as well as support in implementing that advice. It is not a time for sophisticated thinking about complex classroom organization or consideration of a range of teaching strategies. Rather the student teacher may at this stage draw on the professional knowledge of others in order to simplify classroom procedures and achieve at least a small degree of success which can then form the basis for further action. This requires the teacher to articulate her or his own professional knowledge about the nature of that classroom and the teacher and tutor, together, to break down the professional skills required into small enough steps for those to be assimilated and implemented by the student teacher. In this particular case the class teacher was able to do that. However, there is evidence that not all teachers can express the knowledge which they have about their classes and their professional skill (McAlpine *et al.*, 1988). An effective tutor can sometimes act to help teachers articulate that knowledge.

Under these circumstances it would seem that an instructional approach was appropriate at that time. It would require close consultation between teacher, student teacher and tutor in order to ensure that:

- the action which was to be taken was understood by all
- the reasons for the action were also understood
- the implementation was achievable
- there would be appropriate ways for the student teacher to receive feedback.

This rather mechanistic approach would continue only until the student teacher was sufficiently in control of the situation to be able to take a much more proactive role.

Tutor A/student 1

This example was also offered as an illustration of instructional supervision and again the whole context may give clues to the usefulness of the approach.

Student 1 was an extremely competent student teacher working in an excellent team situation with a very supportive class teacher. The tutor in the extract made some very warm evaluative comments about her teaching and then went on to offer some quite specific advice about making folders. It was characteristic of the student teacher that she was extremely thoughtful and well prepared. She consulted with the class teacher almost continuously but more as a colleague than an apprentice. Most of the time they discussed possible teaching strategies and then made decisions about how to act. Up to that time the class teacher had been helping on a regular basis with everyday skills, for example, using a cutter, putting up displays, making workcards and techniques for marking. The student teacher, being very thoughtful indeed, questioned every action she took.

Unlike student 2, it is unlikely that student 1 needed the precise degree of practical help which was being offered to her. On the other hand, she did have the reflective approach which would have enabled her to respond to an invitation to identify her own areas of professional development. There was evidence that she was most anxious to assess the way her classroom was managed and especially the way her own views about this compared and contrasted with those of the class teacher. Because of the very practical everyday nature of their interaction it was not easy for her to develop that sort of reflective dialogue with him. However, such a dialogue involving differences of opinion with the class teacher would have been quite possible in that secure environment and, given the necessary encouragement, the student teacher would almost certainly have identified it as an area for professional development. It could be argued that the tutor may have been more effective by rejecting the instructional role and working to develop a clinical approach.

Alternatively, it would have been possible for the tutor to develop a professional dialogue by taking a more theoretical perspective. Together, they might have identified particular objectives or the theoretical principles underlying a teaching approach and in this way discussed the application of theory in the classroom. This student teacher had enough confidence in what she was doing to be able to use theoretical scrutiny to inform and evaluate her practice.

Tutor D/student 4

This example was offered as an illustration of the development of a professional dialogue using a psychopedagogical approach. Again, the aim of this section is to consider the appropriateness of the approach by examining the context of the school-based work.

Although student 4 had previously had a rather weak block school experience, this time she was functioning very adequately in the classroom. The class teacher was pleased with her work and, in fact, she taught in a similar way to him. Both used a predominantly whole-class approach with very little group work and not a lot of opportunity for practical investigation. Both also had a very personal charismatic style in their handling of the children. The tutor was pleased with the confidence and competence of the student teacher and was anxious to build on that. She felt that the student teacher was competent within the parameters of that classroom, but that she was practising only a narrow range of teaching strategies. In the eyes of the tutor, the result of this was that the student was not extending her teaching skills or developing a reflective approach. The outcome was that, in the judgement of the tutor, the teaching was not as effective as it had the potential to be.

However, because the teacher and student teacher got on so well with each other and because neither really saw any need to change and develop teaching which appeared to be effective, the tutor was faced with the possibility of one of the classical teacher/student teacher/tutor conflicts. In this situation the tutor makes certain suggestions which the teacher and the student teacher ignore, except when the tutor is there! Under these circumstances the tutor used the approach of working as far as possible in a trio (ie, herself working closely with teacher and student teacher), developing a professional dialogue by asking for information about objectives, how the student expected to achieve those and how she would know when she had. She led onto discussion about teaching approaches which would be necessary in order to achieve the stated objectives. The extract gives one example of the results of that discussion, that is the necessary requirements if complex concepts are to be understood and assimilated by children. Because she generated a 'genuine' exchange of ideas and opinions she did not antagonize either student teacher or teacher. At the same time she achieved, at least in part, her own objectives of extending the student teacher's repertoire of teaching approaches.

This example, as well as showing the effective implementation of a psycho-pedagogical approach, also illustrates that the development of this type of professional dialogue will often include the use of instructional techniques, especially when the student teacher, however competent, is using new ideas and the teacher either cannot or does not wish to introduce her or his ideas. To say that some class teachers cannot introduce strategies to student teachers is not the same as saying they cannot use such strategies themselves. It may mean that they are able to teach in that way if they wish but are not able at that time to articulate their actions.

This example contrasts with the one above, student 1. In the latter, it was suggested that either a clinical approach or a psychopedagogical approach would be possible and helpful. In the case of student 4, the psychopedagogical approach seemed to offer the structure which was necessary to promote discussion. Initially, within that context, the need for professional development was not apparent to the teacher and student teacher. An analysis of objectives for learning and the outcomes of learning offered the framework for dialogue.

Tutor C / student 3

In the previous example it was suggested that the professional dialogue would best be achieved by making use of a psychopedagogical approach to supervision with the initiative taken at first by the tutor. On the other hand, for student 1 it was suggested that either approach could be used sensitively to promote professional dialogue. However, there were instances in the research conducted by the writer where a clinical approach would always be preferred. Student 3 was a student whose situation fitted into this category.

Student 3 was a well prepared, creative, professional person who took her teaching and children's learning very seriously. The class teacher with whom she was working also had a strong sense of responsibility to the children she taught. However, the teaching approaches of these two were very different indeed, to the extent that there was a real potential for hostility between them. Because of the initial sensitivity of the tutor and the eventual tolerance and professionalism of all, the difficulties were resolved in an amicable and effective way. However, in the sensitive situation of this block school experience the imposition of a formal theoretical format for discussion could have been counter-productive. At the same time the context itself made such an approach superfluous. In a situation in which two teachers were approaching their teaching in very different ways the potential for appraisal and justification is already built into the classroom context.

Although teacher and student teacher rarely got into a professional dialogue about the strengths and weaknesses of different teaching approaches, they were both concerned about the progress of the children. At the same time the tutor listened to both and ensured that the opinions and perceptions of each were shared. The tutor herself acted as a resource to the student teacher; for example, in the notes she refers to the 'match' between the work set and the children's ability and achievements. The teacher also acted as a resource by listening to the student teacher talk about her plans and her pleasure in the children's achievements.

This illustration provides a strong reminder that supervision is an activity carried out between people and as such should always be responsive to both personal and professional needs.

Implications for Teachers Assuming Responsibility for Training in Schools

It has taken a long time for supervising tutors to learn about effective ways of working with student teachers in school. Most of the development has taken place as tutors have worked more and more closely with teachers and attempted to link the learning which takes place in school with the learning that takes place in the training institutions. In what ways may mentors or teacher-tutors in schools learn from the challenges and pitfalls which tutor supervisors experienced? Three aspects stand out:

- the use of supervision strategies
- the understanding of context
- the value of dialogue.

Each of these will be considered below.

The use of supervision strategies

In the past, some tutors have gone into schools to supervise student teachers without really knowing what they were going to do when they got there. Traditionally, the training programmes for supervising tutors have been minimal. However, over recent years supervision has been taken more seriously. Supervision strategies have been identified, discussed and evaluated. Tutors and teachers have begun to consider such strategies and to decide the roles which each will take in implementing them. The danger now is that teaching is perhaps being seen, once again, as a skill which may be transmitted almost by chance as a teacher and a student teacher happen to be together in the same room. There is a danger of assuming that professional learning will happen just because a student teacher is in school.

However, there is evidence that an understanding of strategies may help mentors just as it does supervising tutors. To be able to identify and describe strategies gives a control over the situation which helps to ensure the best practice. To be able to identify an approach as instruction makes it possible for one to consider first whether that is an appropriate strategy for enhancing student learning and, second, whether one is implementing it in the most effective way.

The understanding of context

Understanding of supervision strategies and skill in implementing them will not be helpful if the strategies are not matched appropriately to contexts. Time and time again, in the research on which this chapter is based, there was evidence of the sensitive and thoughtful ways in which tutors assessed the school contexts in which students were placed. They took account of the skills, attitudes and confidence of the students themselves, the attitudes and support of the cooperating teachers and the many factors in the classroom and school which influenced the conduct of the teaching. The effectiveness of tutors was related to their ability to adapt their supervision behaviour to the circumstances. It became more and more apparent that although knowledge of supervision strategies was very helpful, it was most effective when tutors could adapt that knowledge within context in a reflective way.

Where problems arose they often came about because the tutor had not considered it to be important to access particular information, had underestimated the importance of certain factors, or had made superficial interpretations. Sometimes tutors were not effective because, knowing that they had a lack of understanding of the pressures of a situation, they chose not to act. Their justification was that no action was safer than clumsy action that could aggravate a situation.

Effective tutors had not only a wealth of professional information on which they drew to make judgements, but they were also able to make very good use of case study material from other people. This suggests that teachers involved in teacher training may be able to learn from the professional knowledge of tutors despite the slightly different contexts in which they work. Training in picking up relevant cues will help those teachers make judgements which will enhance their supervision strategies.

The value of dialogue

Like teaching, supervision is a professional skill requiring sensitivity. Those involved differ in their personal qualities and in their professional skills. The introduction outlined some of the difficulties that have been experienced as tutors have tried to work with teachers in the supervision situation. It has been argued that the location of training in schools will somehow be more effective because it will remove these difficulties.

The evidence suggests that this is not the case. Once tutors, teachers and student teachers have developed skills of communication, the interaction within a trio greatly enhances the professional development of student teachers. The aim to develop reflective practice is more likely to be achieved in the uneven interaction of a trio. It is under these circumstances that dialogue takes place because it needs to. The definition of roles, the identification of targets, the evaluation of teaching and children's learning is more effective when agreement is not taken for granted.

References

Cogan, M L (1973) *Clinical Supervision*, Boston: Houghton Mifflin.

Cohn, M M and Gellman, V C (1988) 'A developmental approach for fostering inquiry in pre-service teacher education', *Journal of Teacher Education*, **39**, 2.

Grimmet, P and Ratzloff, H (1986) 'Expectations for the co-operating teacher', *Journal of Teacher Education*, **37**, 6.

McAlpine, A, Brown, S, McIntyre, D and Hagger, H (1988) *Student Teachers Learning from Experienced Teachers*.

Proctor, A (1991) 'Co-operative teaching practice supervision: An analysis of how teachers, student teachers and tutors may work together effectively', unpublished PhD, University of Durham.

Proctor, K A (1993) 'Tutors' professional knowledge of supervision and the implications for supervision practice', in Calderhead, J and Gates, P (eds) *Conceptualizing Reflection in Teacher Development*, London: Falmer Press.

Rust, F O (1988) 'How supervisors think about teaching', *Journal of Teacher Education*, **39**, 2.

Stones, E (1984) *Supervision in Teacher Education*, London: Methuen.

Chapter 11

Mentoring and the Demands of Reflection

Terence H McLaughlin

In recent years there has been much professional and academic discussion of the role of the school-based mentor in initial teacher training (ITT). One of the most prominent features of this discussion has been an insistence that the role of mentor should not be conceived and exercised in narrow or minimalist terms. The mentor is not to be seen as merely a hovering provider of encouragement and vague exhortation, a trainer in routinized skill and knack, or a 'master' whose practice is to be simply emulated. On the contrary, in partnership with institutions of higher education (HEIs), the mentor is seen as having a vital part to play in the wider and deeper aspects of the preparation of teachers, for example in the development of 'the reflective practitioner'. Even when the place of higher education as a partner in fulfilling these broader aims is called into question by colleagues in school (for example, Berrill, 1993; Furlong, 1993) this is not because these aims are seen as irrelevant to the work of the mentor, but because of judgements about the extent to which schools are, or can be, self-sufficient with respect to what is needed.

It is in relation to these 'wider and deeper' aspects of the task of teacher preparation that mentors are likely to experience most uncertainty and anxiety. This is not surprising since what is involved in these aspects is by no means clear. In this chapter I will explore these matters and make some practical observations on these important aspects of the mentor's task.

The chapter has four sections. In the first I indicate major weaknesses in the 'apprenticeship' model of initial training, and in the second I outline a more adequate conception. In the third section I argue that this conception generates an important role for mentors in the development of reflection in student teachers. The demands which this role makes of mentors will be explored in the final section.

Against Narrowness and Minimalism in Initial Teacher Training

'Narrow' and 'minimalist' conceptions of teacher training are familiar enough from recent writing and controversy. Roughly speaking, such conceptions give pride of place to the possession by student teachers of a sound knowledge of the subject to be taught and to the learning of practical teaching skills and competences through experience as an 'apprentice' in school. In some cases, there is hostility towards the value and necessity of training conducted elsewhere than in the school and in particular towards forms of 'theoretical' reflection and study. Such conceptions of training lead naturally to calls for cutting back, and in some cases the elimination of, the participation of HEIs in ITT, and to the relocation of such training in schools.

For good reason, such narrow and minimalist conceptions of training have found little favour among those professionally and academically concerned with teacher training, including those who support a substantial relocation of teacher training in schools on other grounds. Nor have they been accepted by teachers themselves. The profound inadequacy of such conceptions of teacher training is evident. At the heart of this inadequacy is a failure to perceive, let alone give a clear account of, the practical and evaluative complexities inherent in the task of teaching, and the forms of training needed to address them.

For obvious reasons, the task of teaching is unlike making a cake or assembling a car on a production line. In teaching there are no recipes or mechanical procedures to be followed to achieve success. Given the dynamic, complex and unpredictable nature of the classroom, recipes and procedures based on rules are inadequate in the face of the need for flexible 'situational judgement' and appropriate response. Preparation for teaching needs to go beyond such recipes and procedures because successful teaching requires sophisticated technical and strategic judgements and actions which depend upon the teacher possessing forms of knowledge, skills and attitudes which cannot be passed on through crudely conceived forms of school experience alone.

Furthermore educative teaching is inherently value laden. It must be so, since the aims of education involve the development of the person in various respects, and the promotion of that development requires numerous choices and judgements to be made involving values of many kinds. These include judgements about human good which are implicit in general educational ideals and aims, about moral values which are reflected in the aims and processes of education, and about values related to particular areas of the curriculum. The activity of teaching is inescapably evaluative, and teachers must be prepared in such a way that they have a reflectively critical grasp of the matters of value at stake. This is for at least two reasons. First, educational values are the subject of contention and debate. Teachers therefore cannot be merely 'inducted' into a preferred set of values but must be equipped to determine their own position on the questions at issue and engage in professional dialogue about them. Second, the teacher must not only understand the values that he or she is seeking to bring to bear upon learning, but must also 'live' them if they are to bear fruit. They cannot be simply adopted 'second-hand'. These and other reasons give support to the philosopher Israel Scheffler's insistence that educators must be fluent in the evaluation of educational ends as well as means.

What emerges from these considerations is the realization that although 'sitting by Nellie' may be a necessary element in teacher training it is not sufficient unless Nellie is herself charged with, and capable of, introducing students to the broader and deeper requirements of training which have been indicated. Nellie's teaching may well embody flexible situational judgement and be evaluatively rich. But it cannot simply be observed and copied by students if they are to gain all they need to become professional teachers, fully conceived. If the narrow and minimal conception of ITT is rejected, what is the nature of a more adequate account?

Towards an Adequate Conception of Initial Teacher Training

More adequate views of ITT do not reject all the elements of minimalist conceptions or models of training (eg, the emphasis upon practical experience in school) but seek to locate them in a fuller and richer overall account of what is involved in training teachers. Such views typically have three aspects *inter alia*:

(i) an outline of the various logical elements of teaching
(ii) a view of the different elements of training and the forms of expertise and context required for their realization, and
(iii) an account of the nature and scope of critical reflection and assessment in teaching and an indication of how this might be developed in students.

With regard to (i), it is pointed out that teaching requires a number of different kinds of achievement. A teacher must have *knowledge and understanding* of wide-ranging sorts, the ability in the light of that knowledge and understanding to make *rational practical judgements* about what to do in particular circumstances, *skills* to carry out what is decided and *dispositions* (motives and tendencies) to actually do what is judged appropriate (Hirst, 1979). A teacher who is an 'autonomous professional' is able to 'knit together' all these different achievements to produce an effective teaching performance. These different kinds of achievement must therefore be interrelated in training. For example, the various forms of knowledge and understanding which are needed cannot be isolated from the development of the ability to make sound judgements and to exercise skills.

With regard to (ii), a familiar account of the different elements of training is offered by Furlong *et al.* (1988) in their four 'levels' at which it can be conducted:

Level a − *direct practice:* practical training through direct first-hand experience of specific situations in schools and classrooms.
Level b − *indirect practice*: 'detached' training in practical matters usually conducted in classes or workshops within training institutions and not via professional practice itself.
Level c − *practical principles*: critical study of the general principles of practice and their use and justification.
Level d − *disciplinary theory*: critical study of practice and its principles in the light of fundamental theory and research (eg, by reference to the foundation disciplines of education).

These levels are not of course to be seen as wholly separable from each other. Practical principles and disciplinary theory (that is levels c and d) are particularly concerned with the critical and reflective aspects of training which were argued earlier to be vital. But they must be related in a coordinated and carefully planned way to the more 'practical' aspects of training conducted in direct and indirect practice (levels a and b). The training must be integrated in such a way that the student can relate the different elements to each other. The levels are not to be seen as hierarchically related in a crude way, a point obscured to some extent by the use of the term 'levels' rather than, say, 'dimensions'. On the question of the appropriate expertise and context for the realization of these four levels, there is wide agreement that the school, and in particular the mentor, is in a privileged and irreplaceable position to engage in work at level a, although this by no means limits the contribution to training that mentors should make.

With regard to (iii) it is suggested that forms of appropriate critical reflection are central to the notion of the 'autonomous professional'. The need for such reflection is implicit, as we have seen, in the practical and evaluative aspects of the work of the teacher, but is given additional significance through the aspiration to 'professionalism' with its emphasis on expertise which is free from external control. It is only through reflective professional judgement of this kind that educational practice can change and develop. What is needed here is not the sort of reflection required for the academic study of education, but for the professional task of teaching.

Such reflection is, in varying ways, implicit in and necessary to all the interrelated elements outlined in (i) above – the various logical elements in teaching, and (ii) – the different elements of training. At its heart are the insights that it can provide through the analysis, interpretation and explanation of presuppositions and assumptions. While reflection is related to 'the present and the particular' tasks of teaching (it is, after all, reflection for action) it is not limited by, or confined to them. It is in the nature of the reflection envisaged here that it seeks broader frameworks of context, reference and justification, and that it challenges the notion that the 'common sense' of practice is free of judgements, beliefs and values.

The extent to which 'theory' is involved in such reflection has been the subject of much discussion (for example, Hirst, 1990; Smith, 1992). The concept of 'theory' seems to arise naturally once critical reflection gets going. In an attempt to be sensitive, systematic, informed and well grounded, reflection seeks principles and appropriate forms of objectivity and justification. Such concerns are the stuff of theory.

Care is needed in the uncritical use of the term 'theory', for at least two reasons. First, 'theory' can be of many different kinds, ranging from the explicit, articulated and abstract theory contained in the foundation disciplines of education, to the implicit, tacit and intuitive 'practical theory' used by teachers in their daily work. Sensitivity is needed to the particular kind of theoretical reflection that is appropriate for different elements of the training programme, a notion captured in the 'levels' referred to above. Second, in no sense can a programme of training be seen in terms of the *application* of independently learned theory to practice. Rather it is the notion that reflection and 'theorizing' *in* and *from* practice, generating 'practical principles' that is fundamental. It is logically impossible for the foundation disciplines of education alone to provide principles for practice; and it is important to acknowledge and be sensitive to the nature of practical reason itself, that is, the way in which professionals actually think and reflect about their work.

It is in relation to a more adequate conception of ITT of this kind, and the structured programme to which it gives rise, that the role of the mentor should be understood.

Reflection and the Role of the Mentor

In this more adequate model of training it is generally assumed that part of the mentor's work is the development of appropriate forms of reflection in student teachers. It is not yet clear however whether the responsibility of the mentor here is confined to level a of the training programme (encouraging the student to reflect upon experience in a possibly limited way) or whether there is a role for the mentor in developing forms of reflection which include reference to wider issues.

Any suggestion that the role of the mentor should be limited in this way is mistaken. Attention has already been drawn to the way in which all the elements of an adequate model of initial training must be related to each other so that the student can integrate them in his or her professional understanding and practice. For example practice (level a) is seen as inseparable from the critique of that practice through the critical study of general principles (level c), and through engagement with the insights afforded by the foundation disciplines (level d). This has a number of implications for the role of the mentor with regard to reflection.

First there are implications for the way in which the mentor promotes reflection on practice (level a). Reflection is part of this level in an adequate model of training because it involves the development of forms of understanding, judgement and skill and not mere induction into direct practice. But this reflection might be seen as limited in scope. However, if direct practice is inseparable from practical principles and disciplinary theory, the mentor cannot avoid introducing the student to this wider form of reflection from the beginning. The suggestion that reflection can be limited once it is encouraged is mistaken. Wider and more fundamental questions will inescapably arise, even in the early stages of training, and mentors should be aware of this and be prepared to deal with it.

Second, the aim of integrating the various elements of the course clearly would be facilitated by mentors having responsibility not only for training in practice (level a), but also for some of the principles governing that practice in the classroom and the school (level c). It should be remembered that the different aspects of training which the levels subsume do not correspond neatly with a site of training (for example level a only in the school and the other three only in an HEI). There are good reasons on the grounds of integration for the responsibilities of the mentor not to be confined to one level.

A further reason against limiting the role of the mentor in promoting reflection is that he or she will inevitably have a general influence as a person upon students. The significance of this point will be returned to later.

Mentoring and the Demands of Reflection

The claim that the mentor has a responsibility to promote reflection is easy to state. But what demands does this responsibility make upon the mentor? I shall now consider some questions relating to the nature of reflection itself and will conclude with some remarks about the significance of reflection in the context of the role of the mentor as a whole.

The nature of reflection

It is important for mentors to have a clear sense of the *kind* of reflection that it is appropriate for them to promote with student teachers and how to go about it. In the light of points made earlier, it is clearly a mistake to see developing reflection in the student as a matter of applying existing theory to practice in some crude sense. Nor is it a matter of raising complex abstract questions which are not grounded in the demands and realities of practice. Nellie must not be replaced by Socrates! What then is required?

A common answer to this question is that mentors must be concerned with reflection-in-action. Given their privileged access to 'action' it would seem that mentors have a unique role here. However, although discussions of this are thought-provoking (Schon, 1983; 1987) what does the notion actually *mean* in terms of strategies and practices that mentors can adopt? Unless a clear answer can be found to this neglected question, the duty of 'promoting reflection' of the appropriate sort would seem to be a vague slogan. There is therefore an urgent need for work which will assist mentors to achieve an operational sense of what the promotion of reflection-in-action entails. The experience of mentors themselves will make a powerful contribution to such research. Mentors will need to judge whether the notion of 'reflection-in-action', once it is clarified operationally, covers all the forms of reflection they might seek to promote in students; for example, there may be a limited role for the presentation and application of abstract theory.

One of the shortcomings of the notion of 'the reflective practitioner' is that an impression can arise that reflection *in itself* is of value regardless of its outcome. But while students should be encouraged to have the confidence to articulate their perceptions without being unduly concerned, initially at least, about the quality of their deliberations, judgements of the quality of their reflection are in the end inescapable for the mentor. Reflections can be more or less accurate, adequate, insightful, relevant, valid and so forth. Mentors must of course acknowledge that on many issues a number of different points of view are tenable, and they should not be quick to pass premature judgement. But judgement of an appropriate sort by the mentor and indeed by other students on the outcome of reflection cannot be avoided if reflection itself is to have direction and 'bite'. This raises the need for the criteria of judgement invoked by the mentor to be explicit and justifiable in the light of (say) an adequate overall view of the purposes of education.

Although reflection by student teachers takes place all the time, mentors are also confronted with complex judgements concerning the *timing and prioritization* they give to it in a more explicit and formal sense. For example, at what point should a student teacher be invited to reflect upon a teaching skill he or she is struggling to master? Reflection can undermine as well as enhance the development of practical skills. In some cases it might be thought better for student teachers to acquire such skills in a rather uncritical way at first, and then submit them to reflection later. Such matters need to be carefully judged by mentors.

Questions also arise about the *extent* of reflection that should be encouraged. These are in part related to the degree of involvement of the mentor in the various levels of training discussed earlier. There is no reason in principle why mentors should not promote reflection at level d of the training course, where reference is made to the educational disciplines in order to illuminate practical teaching, granted that what is done fits into a coherent overall programme. Questions of the validity of the reflection generated need to be borne in mind here however, together with the related need for expertise and training in the relevant forms of educational disciplinary theory. The mere raising of questions is insufficient. Engagement by students in some detail with a range of coherent answers is necessary. This point illustrates the need for forms of mentor training to be wide-ranging in scope, and not confined to matters of technique and strategy. A failure to provide this will limit the capacity of mentors to assume fuller responsibilities in other levels of training.

Another issue which arises for mentors in relation to the promotion of reflection can be described as the possibility of *contextual conflict*. There is an important difference between the sort of critical reflection which takes place in a university seminar, where students can discuss matters in the abstract, and that which takes place in the context of a particular school. In the latter, it may be difficult to separate judgement and criticism of (say) teaching strategies and policies from judgement and criticism of the particular members of staff responsible for them. The possibility of the inhibition of critical reflection in school by factors of diplomacy and embarrassment is one which mentors must confront. The limitations of merely abstract discussion of matters of educational practice has long been recognized, but possible limitations and difficulties relating to critical reflection in the school context require equal recognition and appropriate remedy.

In order to achieve aims such as these, the mentor must possess the qualities and capacities of critical reflection applied to education and (in the light of the next section) life itself. These are only in part intellectual. For example, a reflective mentor will necessarily engage in the practice of challenging 'edu-babble' (imprecise and platitudinous rhetoric applied to education) and will also ask critical questions about the meaning and adequacy of concepts such as 'competence' in teaching. This requires not only relevant forms of understanding on the part of the mentor, but also a disposition not to be taken in by slogans which have a surface meaning and plausibility but which are in need of careful analysis.

The place of reflection in the overall role of the mentor

The promotion of appropriate forms of reflection is only one of the tasks of the mentor. Apart from practical training, the mentor must provide support and encouragement to student teachers and develop in them qualities of the professional teacher in addition to reflection. These include personal qualities and virtues such as distance, humility, courage, impartiality, open-mindedness, empathy, enthusiasm and imagination (Hare, 1993). Mentors must also act as 'models' to student teachers for the full range of qualities of a professional teacher, including broad human spirit and sympathy. Reflection is only one of these qualities and it is clear that the influence of the mentors depends as much upon the sort of person they are in general as upon any reflective capacity they may possess or seek to develop in their students.

Reflection and the capacity to promote it in student teachers nevertheless hold an important place in the qualities of the mentor. Without appropriate reflection, the other qualities of the teacher or mentor may be directed to inadequate or misguided educational goals. It can be plausibly argued that one of the most powerful elements of the example set by a mentor is the embodiment of a form of wisdom, rooted in and revealing commitment to a broad and rich grasp of the values of the educational enterprise (Smith and Alred, 1993). This cannot be reduced to, but requires, precisely the sort of appropriate reflection that it has been argued is the duty of the mentor to promote.

References

Berrill, M (1993) 'It's time we were frank', *Times Educational Supplement*, 8 January.

Furlong, J (1993) 'Why wear blinkers?', *Times Educational Supplement*, 29 January.

Furlong, J, Hirst, P, Pocklington, K and Miles, S (1988) *Initial Teacher Training and the Role of the School*, Buckingham: Open University Press.

Hare, W (1993) *What Makes a Good Teacher*, Canada: Althouse Press.

Hirst, P (1979) 'Professional studies in initial teacher education', in Alexander, R and Wormald, E (eds) *Professional Studies for Teaching*, Guildford: Society for Research in Higher Education.

Hirst, P (1990) 'The theory practice relationship in teacher training', in Booth, M, Furlong, J and Wilkin, M (eds) *Partnership in Initial Teacher Training*, London: Cassell.

Schon, D (1983) *The Reflective Practitioner*, London: Basic Books.

Schon, D (1987) *Educating the Reflective Practitioner*, San Francisco, CA: Jossey-Bass.

Smith, R (1992) 'Theory: an entitlement to understanding', *Cambridge Journal of Education*, 22, 3.

Smith, R and Alred, G (1993) 'The impersonation of wisdom', in McIntyre, D, Hagger, H and Wilkin, M (eds) *Mentoring: Perspectives on school-based teacher education*, London: Kogan Page.

Chapter 12

Quality Assurance

William Taylor

The Quality Movement

The discussion of quality in education ought to be about making people happier, more effective, more creative, more fulfilled. Sadly, it often isn't. After ten years of sitting high on the educational agenda, quality as idea and as process is in danger of becoming bureaucratized and boring.

Library shelves and journal racks grown under the weight of portentous definitions, analyses and assertions concerning quality. The conference circuit resonates with hortatory utterances about the importance of personal and institutional commitments to quality. The range of educational acronyms has been much extended by the setting up of bodies responsible for quality control, quality audit, quality assurance, quality improvement, quality care and quality management. Institutions find themselves playing host to one review team after another and having to prepare increasingly complex justifications for their objectives, internal organization, course design and delivery and how they evaluate the outcomes of their efforts. As the controversies over pupil assessment have shown, the assessment of quality can become highly politicized.

Where did all this come from and why does it matter to those in schools, universities and colleges who are today concerned with developing new forms of collaborative teacher education?

It is easy – too easy – to conclude that education is suffering from the importation by trade-balance-obsessed politicians of ideas and practices originally developed to enhance competitiveness and profitability in the industrial sphere. True, in industry and commerce the terms quality control, quality assurance and quality management have come to signify not just important practical processes and techniques, but expansionist inspirational movements. The gurus who exemplify the movement, its philosophers who

---

write the exemplary texts, its practitioner saints, holy sites, creeds, commandments and proverbs are increasingly visible.

The quality movement, like all others, seeks converts. Individuals and organizations are enjoined to renounce their evil ways – unclear goals, waste, short-term profitability at the expense of customer satisfaction, shoot-from-the-hip management, indifference to market trends, dependence on protectionism and the welfare ethic, resistance to competition. By total immersion in the quality ethic, they will be born again to the virtues of mission statements, strategic thinking, customer closeness and care, right first time, nil defect, formative evaluation and continuous improvement.

How does – how *should* – teacher education stand in relation to this movement?

Quality and Values

From the beginning, there have been cautions about the extent to which ideas about quality can or should be applied to education. Students are not just 'consumers' or 'customers'. The teacher-student relationship is much more than a one-way provision of goods and services. Education should not simply satisfy the expectations of employers, parents and pupils; it should help to *redefine* their expectations. Research in universities and colleges is not a production-line activity; new knowledge cannot be produced to order. Much of what teachers do is subject to influence by social and personal factors outside their control, and for which they cannot be held accountable – and so on.

Such cautions are understandable and justified. Inevitably, they have also been used to defend entrenched provider interests. Seen thus, they have provoked impatience, and not only on the part of governments of radical persuasion. In the words of a recent report of the Australian Higher Education Council (1992) on *Achieving Quality*:

> A higher education system that justly prides itself on its deep analysis of issues
> of consequence is sometimes strangely reluctant to examine its own processes
> equally deeply, publicly and comprehensibly, and without rancour.

Fortunately, most educators now recognize that the quality movement in education represents something much deeper than a simple infection of universities and schools by politically-motivated ideas culled from the world of work.

Civil society at the end of the twentieth century requires the reconciliation of interests that are increasingly plural, visible and vocal. There is less deference to 'professionals'. The demystification of institutions and of knowledge, for which the radical left long campaigned, has been taken up by the radical right. Individuals and organizations placed in positions of authority must be willing to justify their actions. In particular, any decision that results in an individual or group being treated *differently* must be based on publicly available criteria – something that has led resource distributing agencies to create a plethora of performance measures and outcome indicators.

The ability of societies to trade successfully in an increasingly global market place, to exploit what competitive advantages by way of raw materials, skill and knowledge they possess, and thus to provide employment for their populations, depends heavily on the success of educational systems. None of these things are inimical to what are often identified as *educational* values. The identification of such values as in some way different from (and explicitly or by implication superior to) economic, social and political values has bedevilled too many debates about education in recent years.

Concerns about quality are here to stay. They are not the property of any one ideological or power group. They are likely to survive any conceivable change of government. The quality project has many roots and embraces many different and sometimes inconsistent purposes.

'Quality' begs many questions – to define it as 'fitness for purpose' is useful when legitimizing differences in provision, but does nothing to resolve long-standing debates about the purposes themselves. An emphasis on quality demonstrates the effects of democratization, openness and participation; the importance of public accountability; the continuing value of extending educational opportunities and identifying and nurturing talent, irrespective of its social origins. At the same time, it has been prayed in aid to justify early selection for academic education, a stronger vocational orientation in mass secondary schooling and the need to strengthen national economic advantage.

It follows that we need to be sensitive to and prepared to be critical about the assumptions and common sense understandings that underlie the application of quality concepts to any particular educational activity – if you like, to the *theories* of the field. Such criticism, it must be emphasized, should not be seen merely as a way of exposing, as some educators of the left have tried to do, the exploitative capitalist values that permeate such activity. Nor is it a means to defend the traditional disciplines of knowledge and personal conduct of which the educational right sees itself as the guardian.

It is a great pity that the word 'critical' has been appropriated by the left and consequently demonized by the right. To understand and be critical of our beliefs and assumptions about curriculum, character and society, to be clear about what is involved in the processes of learning and teaching, is a responsibility that all teachers share.

Choices and decisions that enhance the quality of education can only be made on the basis of critical understanding. The quality movement needs to be approached in the same analytical and sceptical spirit as any other development. If after careful investigation it turns out to be consistent with worthwhile values, to have within it the means of securing desirable ends, and not to have a downside of unintended consequences that might wipe out whatever gains it might confer, then it deserves our willing – but never uncritical – support.

Quality in teacher preparation

While it is the measures to control and improve the quality of initial teacher preparation introduced since about 1980 that will determine the agenda for the next few years, these recent developments can only be properly understood in the context of what went before.

Nineteenth century efforts to maintain quality included a national curriculum for teacher preparation and close supervision of the work of self-standing training colleges (established by the churches and voluntary bodies) by members of Her Majesty's Inspectorate, which itself had been set up in 1839. After 1902, local education authorities were able to fund their own colleges and an increasing proportion of secondary teachers began to receive professional training in university departments of education. In the mid-1920s boards were established to examine the students of colleges grouped together round a local university, and after the report of an official committee (known as the McNair Report) at the end of the Second World War these developed into 'Area Training Organizations' (ATOs).

During the 35 years of the ATOs' existence, certificate, diploma and, later, degree level work was subject to scrutiny and approval by the academic bodies of the universities with which the colleges were affiliated, a process known as validation. HMI continued to play a role in reporting on courses and institutional provision. Representatives of teachers and local authorities sat on the professional committees and councils of the ATOs responsible for examining and recommending recognition of students' professional competence. Colleges and departments sought reports from the staff of the schools in which students carried out periods of practice teaching. Examiners from other institutions saw students at work in classrooms and scrutinized their written assignments and examination scripts. Much of this scrutiny related to who should pass and at what level. Judgements were based on individual performance, not on overall course quality.

With the decision in the mid-1970s to integrate teacher education into the 'binary system' of universities and polytechnics that had been developing over the previous ten years, and the virtual disappearance of single-purpose training institutions, the ATOs lost their role. Many of the new multi-purpose colleges sought validation of their awards not from a university but from the Council for National Academic Awards (CNAA), which had been established to award degrees in non-university institutions of higher education. From its beginnings the CNAA had been required to establish and maintain quality standards equivalent to those of universities. In order to do so, and to be *seen* to be doing so, it developed systematic, explicit and bureaucratic codes of practice and procedures for the maintenance of quality. As a result, polytechnics and colleges were in some respects in better shape than the then universities to respond to the quality movement of the 1980s.

Many of the characteristics of quality control, quality audit and quality assurance in teacher education today have been influenced by this history. What is new is the recognition that good buildings, well-endowed libraries, highly qualified staff and first class facilities do not *in themselves* guarantee high quality outcomes. They can only do so in the context of the individual and institutional commitments that go to make up a quality culture.

The involvement of teacher education in the modern quality movement can be said to have begun in 1982 with a paper written by Her Majesty's Inspectorate for the Advisory Committee on the Education and Training of Teachers (ACSET), the proposals in which (via the White Paper *Teaching Quality*) formed the basis for the establishment in 1984 of the Council for the Accreditation of Teacher Education (CATE). In that year CATE began the detailed scrutiny of courses against published criteria issued by the Secretary of State, taking into account reports on institutions prepared by HMI.

Pressures on the public purse, a concern for greater economy, efficiency and effectiveness in educational provision, and the need for funding bodies to be able to justify giving some institutions more money than others, led in the mid-1980s to universities and colleges being prodded and pushed into setting up more explicit and visible quality mechanisms than had existed hitherto.

Now that teacher preparation and development are becoming a collaborative partnership between schools and HEI, the overall quality requirements will apply as much to the school-based and school-led components of training as to those which take place in universities. This is no small matter. With the recent abolition of the CNAA and the redesignation as universities of the polytechnics and some large colleges, there is now in excess of 100 separate institutions with degree-granting powers. Applying quality requirements to such a number is a large but not unmanageable task. But in teacher education the new approach requires the active participation of the managements and staffs of several *thousand* separate schools. How can this be done in a way that contributes to the improvement of teacher education yet does not generate an intolerable degree of bureaucratization?

Definitions and mechanisms

Most institutions take their approach to quality from the 1989 White Paper on Higher Education, which defines *quality control* as the in-house means for maintaining and enhancing quality; *quality audit* as the external mechanism for ensuring that suitable means of quality control are in place and working; and *quality assessment* as the process of externally reviewing and making judgements on teaching and learning in institutions.

Thus quality control is a task for the HEIs themselves. Many have set up quality standards committees or boards and have promulgated detailed codes of practice dealing with such matters as internal validation and review of course structure and content; reporting lines and accountability; consistency and comparability in assessment procedures; the selection, appointment and role of internal and external examiners; the monitoring of individual progress; and course revision and development. Collaboration and partnership with schools requires that heads and teachers play a full part in these processes. Where a consortium of schools is funded to undertake training, it will be directly responsible for quality to the accreditation and funding bodies concerned.

As things stand, overall responsibility for institutional quality audit rests with the university-owned and London-based Higher Education Quality Council (HEQC). This has taken over some of the functions of the former Academic Assessment Unit originally set up by the Committee of Vice Chancellors and Principals, and some of those of the former CNAA. The HEQC has three divisions. One looks after the audit of institutions' quality control mechanisms; another deals with credit accumulation and access courses; the third focuses on the enhancement of quality through staff development and related means.

Institutions must satisfy the HEQC on their mechanisms for quality control in respect of awards made to teachers – bachelor of education and other first degrees that carry teaching qualifications, post graduate certificates of education, advanced diplomas and higher degrees in education – in just the same way as for awards in other subjects and professional fields.

External assessment of the quality of teaching and learning in HEIs is the task of the Higher Education Funding Councils for England and Wales (HEFC[E] and HEFC[W]). The outcome of such assessment, in terms of the three categories of excellent, satisfactory and unsatisfactory, affects institutional funding. So, of course, do the judgements that the funding councils make of institutions' research performances in the course of a four-yearly exercise that began in the mid-1980s. Research quality in each subject area – including education – is graded and the outcomes published. Inevitably, journalists and others have summed and averaged the grades awarded as measures of overall institutional quality, something that neither the funding councils nor the universities themselves encourage.

A few years ago, it was proposed that universities should be classified in three categories in terms of the scale and quality of their research and funded accordingly. Although this idea has been dropped, there is now a *de facto* classification on the basis of differential funding consequent upon the outcomes of the research grading and teaching quality assessments. As a result, some HEIs have less money to play with than others. This has influenced their negotiations with schools about the transfer of funds in support of the school-based elements of initial training under the DfE's 1992 and 1993 teacher training circulars.

Concerns have been expressed about the impact on institutions of the separate HEQC and HEFC review processes. In the case of teacher education, CATE's reviews and, through the new Office of Standards in Education (OfSTED), those of HMI have also had to be reckoned with. Hence fears in some quarters about bureaucratization.

After one false start – the HEFC ITT assessment exercise for 1993/4 was abandoned after it was found that the available evidence did not allow reliable judgements about quality to be made – the HEFCs and OfSTED sought to minimize the burden on institutions by establishing a common inspection and assessment process. As a first step, institutions were to prepare a self-assessment on the basis of a 'template' with six sections. The first of these required a statement of the institution's aims and objectives, with evidence of how these were being met. The second asked for profiles of student entries and their progression. The third had to do with the quality of teaching and learning, including their relation to research, the use made of external advice in devising and implementing courses, employability, and methods of internal course evaluation. The fourth called for information on staff numbers, qualifications, experience and development, the fifth dealt with physical resources and learning support facilities, and the final section was about academic management and quality control.

In the case of ITT it was further suggested that the self-assessments should include details of how courses were accredited; how the competencies required under the Secretary of State's criteria were developed; how subject studies were delivered and relevance to the National Curriculum and appropriate school focus secured; how students are provided with a variety of learning opportunities and experiences through the selection of partner schools; how consistency in assessment was maintained; what arrangements were made for training and deploying school-based mentors; and how responsibility for quality control and enhancement was shared between institutions and their partner schools. All this had to be squeezed into ten pages (font and point size unspecified!) but further contextual background information can be provided by a statistical profile.

The school-based reforms of teacher education are being introduced on a phased basis. The secondary circular was issued in mid-1992 and that relating to primary training not until more than a year later. Thus the first round of HEFC/OfSTED reports was to relate only to providers of secondary courses. Those for primary providers were not due to start until January 1995.

Of the 11 academic subject categories (ASCs) designated by the HEFC(E), the ITT element of the education ASC was to be unique in that the review would be organized and implemented by OfSTED. The HMI members of each OfSTED team were to be joined by an assessor recruited by the HEFC(E), who might be from an HEI *or a school*. The different systems of course and institutional grading that OfSTED and HEFC(E) have used hitherto would be integrated. Details of the methods to be employed by each team were to be included in a draft inspection handbook to be issued for consultation in late 1993.

Even before the outcomes of consultation on its proposals for making primary teacher training more school-based had been made known, ministers put forward a scheme of school-centred (or what might more accurately be described as *school-provided*) teacher education. This decreed that the funds hitherto distributed to universities and colleges in support of initial training, higher degrees and some aspects of educational research by the HEFC(E) should in future be channelled through a newly created Teacher Training Agency (TTA). One of the functions of the agency would be to encourage consortia of schools to bid for ITT funds, thus extending the small-scale school-centred scheme that had been initiated in the Spring of 1993. These consortia would contract with HEI to provide aspects of teacher preparation that could not be offered from their own resources, such as subject studies for the BEd degree.

In a section of the document entitled 'Ensuring Quality', two options were set out for comment. The first retained the basis of institutional accreditation advanced in Circular 9/92, with qualified teacher status being awarded to all successful graduates of courses approved by the Secretary of State. The second would require the TTA to control quality through funding. Providers of training would need to satisfy the agency that quality criteria were met as a condition for future support.

The politicization of teacher education in recent years makes it likely that disputes about organization, control and funding will continue for some time. It seems doubtful, however, if there is any going back on the principle of closer and more equal collaboration between schools and HEI, or on the priority of assuring quality. Future arrangements for the funding and accreditation of teacher education are likely to feature many of the elements of quality assurance worked out by the Funding Councils, CATE, OfSTED and the HEQC in 1992/3.

Such quality assurance depends today on attitudes, practices and procedures that are largely independent of particular reporting and auditing arrangements. Whatever form the latter may take in future, schools and HEI will need to establish what can usefully be called a *quality culture*.

Collaborative quality cultures

Once upon a time teacher education was mainly a task for small training colleges catering largely for 18-year old entrants, or university departments of education recruiting recent graduates. Courses were of common length and standard pattern, reflecting unspoken but widely accepted agreement about pedagogy, curriculum content and expected outcomes. Syllabuses were often skeletal, meetings minimal, assessments informal. Today, much less can be taken for granted. Any and everything can be challenged. And paper work, academic organization and institutional management are complex and time-consuming.

Such bureaucratization is in part a consequence of the participative styles that accompany democratization and the decline of deference. It is in part due to the absence of an accepted canon in many disciplines and professional studies – and it is in part a means whereby individuals and organizations protect themselves against challenges by rejected applicants, disgruntled students, contract-conscious colleagues, accountability-aware funding bodies, corridor-wise practitioners, anxious administrators and point-scoring politicians.

The education of a teacher today does not start on registration day at a HEI or school consortium and end with the award of qualified teacher status. It is a multi-stage process which encompasses recruitment; selection; subject studies at a level appropriate to higher education; pre-service professional and pedagogical studies and practice; certification; induction; a variety of forms of in-service education and training (INSET), including further subject and professional studies and preparation for specialist roles in such fields as curriculum leadership, special needs, and educational management. The requirements of quality assurance, assessment, audit and enhancement apply at each and every one of these stages of a career-long process of continuous professional development. Clear objectives, systematic planning, closely monitored implementation, objective evaluation and active review need to characterize every stage of teacher education.

School-based and school-centred initial training are not just a matter of extending students' periods of teaching practice. They require that all those involved in advancing subject knowledge and developing professional skills play a part in recruiting and selecting students, designing and delivering courses and assessing competence. There is no blueprint for how this should be done. The agencies responsible for ensuring the quality of ITT state entry requirements and set out the overall structure of courses in terms of length, balance of subject and professional studies, minimum time to be spent in the classroom and competences to be achieved, but this still requires many of the most important decisions to be made by those who design and organize courses and teach and assess students.

Such decisions relate to the selection of able, appropriately motivated students; the appointment and deployment of staff who are well-qualified academically and by previous experience to undertake the higher education and professional training of young – and not so young – adults; the provision of books and equipment and IT resources adequate to meet the teaching and learning needs of such students and staff; the identification, organization and acquisition of those facts, concepts, ideas and skills that a student needs to meet the initial competence criteria and to have a basis for sound practice and continuing personal and professional development; and the assessment and evaluation of such knowledge and skill.

In the context of collaborative school-based or school-centred training, it is useful to identify the kinds of activities and behaviours on the part of students and staff that all this requires and the places where it occurs.

Broadly speaking, the things that students *do* in initial training can be summarized as looking, listening, reading, writing, discussing and practising. The last of these involves not only the teaching of individual pupils, groups and whole classes, but participation in those other activities that are part of a teacher's professional responsibilities, such as curriculum planning, pastoral care, assessment and relating to parents. The *places* in which these things are done include classrooms, other school spaces, seminar rooms, libraries, laboratories and students' own rooms at home, in residences or in lodgings.

Effective collaborative training involves many more people and many more sites than the largely institution-based work that it replaces. What was previously the responsibility of 90 or so HEI becomes the shared task of several thousand separate schools, and may also involve HEI that have no previous experience as providers of ITT. In these circumstances the establishment and maintenance of quality could become an even more complex – and bureaucratized – task than at present. Such an outcome is inconsistent with the philosophy that has driven many recent changes, not just in education, but in many other areas of public policy.

This philosophy emphasizes the importance of breaking producer monopolies by diversifying sources of supply; empowering the consumer and improving feedback *to* and the responsiveness *of* providers; reducing central costs and devolving more responsibility to directly accountable operating units. Importantly for our present purposes, inspection and rejection are meant to be replaced by *designed-in quality*.

This last point is vital to the success of innovative forms of initial teacher preparation and for avoiding the bureaucratization that will otherwise be associated with a proliferation of providers. It is the quality of what students see, hear, read, write, think about, say and perform that determines the effectiveness of teacher education. The crucial questions about quality have to do with who is selected for training; what is specified in syllabuses; the books and journals that are read; the lectures and suggestions and seminar contributions that are heard and cogitated upon; the concepts and ideas that help to shape perception, generate reflection and debate and underpin professional understanding; and the skills that are developed in contact with practitioners who not only exemplify high standards but can communicate to the unconfident beginner what is involved in delivering what long experience has made to seem an effortless performance.

Building in quality in an educational setting means providing the conditions in which appropriately qualified and experienced individuals can be imbued with commitments to achieve the highest academic and professional standards of which they are capable. There is an old saying that honesty is the best policy, but he or she who lives by that maxim is not an honest person. Audits, assessments and appraisals of quality should not be the focus of individual or of institutional interest and concern. What matters is that every lecture, every lesson, every laboratory session, every seminar, every essay, every seminar contribution, should be subject to stringent, self-imposed criteria of relevance and of success by staff and students alike.

Individual staff and students cannot deliver quality on the basis of reading and signing up to nationally and locally produced standards, useful as these may be. There are many things that cannot be learned from a textbook; quality is one of them. The real value to staff of the codes of practice, lists of desired outcomes, syllabuses, competency criteria, reading requirements and all the other paraphernalia produced by course teams within departments and other academic units, scrutinized by curriculum development groups, approved by faculties and validated by senates (or their local equivalents) is not the outcome in terms of neatly bound and properly authorized documents, but the educative effects of the process by which these documents were produced.

School-centred training requires the involvement in such processes of all those who are going to be concerned with teaching students and assessing their work in classroom, seminar room or laboratory. Somehow, time will have to be found for school-based mentors and serving teachers to think through the what, the how and the where of developing teaching competence. Documents presented to the TTA or the HEFC(E) or the HEQC or OfSTED or whatever will only carry conviction as an assurance of quality if they reflect the outcome of processes in which all those concerned with a course or a programme of study have taken part, and which have helped to incorporate appropriate quality standards into the consciousness and the consciences of individuals.

This can only happen if the right people are chosen to educate and induct teachers. This is not a task for heads and governors to assign to members of staff who are senior and experienced enough to expect promotion, but who have fallen short of the standards required or have failed in competition. Given the current balance of straight-from-school and mature entrants to teaching, some students will be older than those appointed as their mentors. There are good classroom teachers who are not good at working with adults and there are good classroom teachers who like working with adults but who do not find it easy to analyse their own teaching activities and to communicate knowledge and skills to beginners. As other contributions to this book make clear, the selection and training of mentors is not as simple as some advocates of school-centred training have made it seem.

Systematic staff development is an essential feature of any quality culture. Many HEIs have appointed staff with sole responsibility for such work. Since those responsible for teacher education within school-centred consortia are likely to remain in the employment of their separate schools, the future organization of staff development will require a good deal of sympathetic inter-school coordination.

A collaborative structure for designing, scrutinizing, approving and reviewing the content and pedagogy of teacher education, the designation of roles such as mentor and professional tutor, and the preparation and presentation of documents that lend credence to claims for successful outcomes, are only the visible manifestations of a much more important process. That process needs to have as its aim the creation of a culture within which every member of staff and every student is aware of the standards required, has the means and the motivation to achieve those standards, cares about falling short, and is committed to continuous personal and professional development.

However onerous and eagle-eyed, close external supervision and bureaucratic control will never succeed in raising levels of teacher performance and pupil achievement and in contributing to a prosperous economy, a harmonious polity and a just society unless they engage and enhance the willing and enthusiastic commitment to quality of teachers themselves. The collaborative forms of teacher education and training now being developed must meet that challenge if they are to be judged as successful.

References

Australian Higher Education Council, National Board of Employment (1992) *Achieving Quality*, Canberra: Australian Government Publishing Service.

Chapter 13

The Year 2000

Richard Pring

Introduction: Financial and Political Background

There are about 90 institutions of higher education involved in teacher education, catering for 46,000 students. It is one of the largest and therefore most expensive sectors of higher education, especially as over a half of the trainees are on four-year courses. Furthermore, there are immense hidden costs which have, with few exceptions, never been acknowledged. I refer to the costs to schools of supporting these students, until now without any financial compensation.

The present system, therefore, cannot survive. First, the expansion of higher education in the last three years can be only at the expense of the unit of resource – higher education, including professional training, must become cheaper per capita, unless there is an economic miracle which enables the Treasury to be more generous. Second, the schools, now operating increasingly like small businesses and conscious of the performance indicators by which they will be judged, will understandably seek compensation for the cost of whatever contribution they make to teacher training or indeed to any other activity which is not their prime concern. Higher education, therefore, must necessarily feel the squeeze – less money to do its job and more money to pay out to those to whom so much of the work has in effect been franchised. The future must take into account these financial realities.

The political context also forces higher education to reconsider its future. The widespread criticism (often politically inspired and contrary to the evidence) of schools and their teachers inevitably rebounds on those who have trained the teachers. Thus, if schools are failing, it would seem right to put some of the blame for failure upon the training institutions themselves. Poor teaching presupposes (though not logically) poor training. That thesis, propounded in many places, is two-fold. First, teacher training, in being beguiled by theory, has failed to train for practice. It is as though trainers have taken seriously the advice of Dr Jackson of Exeter College, Oxford, and the first Principal of the Oxford University Day Training College:

> Universities should provide for courses on theory and the half-fledged teachers should thus be scattered to the schools where arrangements for practical training should be made, this being no concern of the University lecturers in theory (Bryce Report, 1895, pp.vi, 205).

They have taken this advice seriously (so it is believed) by indulging in theory and failing to teach the practice: how to organize classrooms, teach reading, keep discipline, 'scattering them' instead to the schools. Furthermore (again, so it is argued) this is inevitable where the difference between theory and practice is institutionalized.

The second aspect of the purported poor training, following the separation of theory from practice, lies in the nature of the theory. That theory is seen to be the wrong sort of theory, one which has created a generation of child-centred practice. In this John Dewey and those who draw upon his work are seen to be the chief perpetrators of a false philosophy, one which focuses upon the growing interests of the child rather than upon the subject matter to be learnt (irrespective of these interests), one which equates learning with growth rather than with the systematic acquisition of knowledge, and one which shifts responsibility from the individual to the social environment.

The financial squeeze and the political scepticism together bode ill for the future of higher education in the training of teachers. They bode ill particularly if those in universities and in colleges simply dismiss the charges as though there is no element of truth in them.

Historical Lesson

It is important to be reminded of how the present situation was reached. It has not always been the case that teachers have been trained or felt the need for training. Also submitting evidence to the Bryce Commission in 1895, Herbert Warren, President of Magdalen College, Oxford, argued that the student who has read Plato's *Republic* and Aristotle's *Politics* and *Ethics* has whatever theory is necessary for the practice of teaching, although in addition it would be helpful

> that a young man who has passed through an English public school, more particularly if he has been ... a prefect ... has had experience in keeping order

and maintaining discipline. ... Thus the average Oxford man, more especially the classical student, ought not to require so long an additional training, either in theory or practice, as is sometimes necessary for students elsewhere (Bryce Report, 1895, pp.v, 257).

Such a belief has persisted and many private schools still recruit staff from those who have demonstrated through prowess on the sports field or through excellence at the university that they have something distinctive to offer young people. Only character and personality are the extra ingredients required and those will not arise from teacher training courses.

What persuaded the dons of Oxford in 1895 that more was required than a public school education was, in the words of Mr Sidgwick of Corpus:

> that the training of teachers *as a whole* was the business of the University and should consist not only in the theory and history of education but also in instruction in the practice of teaching and in an apprentice to schools in some relationship with the University (Bryce Report, 1895, pp.241–2).

The history of teacher training this century has been a history of that – of getting right the relationship of the theory of education with the practice of teaching, and of the apprenticeship to schools with the relationship to the university. It is not right yet. But where could and where should it be by the year 2000?

One problem has certainly been the search for academic respectability in a manner which is normally associated with universities, namely in the creation of a body of knowledge supported by a tradition of scholarship and research. But the connection of this with the practice of teaching was not always made clear to those who were learning to practise. It was as though theory should precede practice, as though a theoretical perspective would illuminate and improve practice. Certainly for many years it was often thought necessary, if not sufficient, to expose the trainee teachers to the thoughts of the great educators, to Plato's *Republic* and to Rousseau's *Emile*. But this was questioned in the 1960s – the 'undifferentiated mush', as RS Peters called it at the 1964 Hull Conference of the Association of Teachers in Colleges and Departments of Education, too often passed for theory. It was necessary, so it was argued, to bring the same academic discipline to bear upon educational studies as it was upon any other area of professional training. Thus were established within university departments the 'foundation disciplines' of educational studies – the philosophy and the sociology of education alongside the psychology and the history which had always been there.

Within a brief time, professional degrees were established; first the ordinary three-year BEd, then the four-year honours BEd. The theoretical perspectives within the foundation disciplines generated their own controversies, producing thereby a subject matter which could be the basis of academic and intellectual study by a graduate profession.

But now it is this which is questioned, questioned both as a suitable basis for professional practice and as academically respectable in its own right. Such questioning has been around a long time and there is therefore inevitably a long academic debate on whether there is such a discipline as educational theory. The philosopher DJ O'Connor (1957) argued that there can be no such thing as educational theory, a claim that is echoed in so much of the destructive criticism of university involvement in teacher training.

O'Connor's argument was as follows. Theory is a systematic set of propositions which describes, explains and predicts what will happen. For example, a learning theory would *descriptively* do justice to a wide range of transactions which take place between teacher and pupil; it would give a coherent explanation of why and in what circumstances certain sorts of learning took place and others did not; and it would be able to predict what teaching activities would be successful. Furthermore, such a clear theoretical account would be open to falsification – when, for example, the child does not learn.

However, O'Connor continued, there simply are not these clear, well tested and falsifiable sets of propositions. There are but two sorts of statement – those expressing desirable goals to be pursued, such as knowledge and understanding (or vague ones like personal growth and maturity), and those concerned with the right steps for reaching those ends, that is empirical and falsifiable statements about the best means to a chosen end. With regard to the first sort of statements, these reflect desires and wishes and are of no theoretical significance. With regard to the second, they require a theory of method – a body of knowledge which, having been acquired, would guide the teacher in teaching mathematics to 10-year-olds or in putting across the complexities of atomic theory to undergraduates. But, says O'Connor, there is no such theory. If there were, then our classrooms would have been transformed by such illumination. Hence, concludes O'Connor, educational theory is but a courtesy title given to a disconnected set of facts, principles, norms, slogans, prescriptions – and to common sense.

O'Connor wrote this 35 years ago. But the arguments prevail in important and influential places. Combined with the financial pressures, they help undermine the argument for preserving a university involvement in teacher training. In the absence of relevant theory, teachers must learn from practice. Furthermore, in keeping with a more general move towards assessment-driven learning, represented by the National Council for Vocational Qualifications, 'good practice' is broken down into a finite list of competences – the 'can dos' which can be observed (or, in the failing apprentice, not observed) and ticked off. Teaching is essentially a matter of acquiring skills and good practice, not a matter of learning theory or developing a theoretical perspective. The Council for the Accreditation of Teacher Education (CATE), in accrediting teacher training departments through a list of performance indicators relating to the Secretary of State's approved competences, may have looked as though it were no more than giving a nudge in a particular direction to university departments – tightening up, as it were, an operation which had become a little slack. But in effect it was much more than that. It was imposing a way of thinking, an anti-theoretical stance, a mode of operating which could brook no critical encounter of the kind that universities stood for and which confirmed O'Connor's deepest suspicions. The theory had been the emperor's clothes, and once it was seen not to exist, then the consequences were obvious – a switching of power and of money to those who practise. The suggestion is that the schools should buy back from universities particular services with their new found money. But, of course, denied the regular and predictable income, the university departments will not be there to be bought into.

This anti-theory, anti-intellectualism is, of course, part of the shifting language of education, exemplified in a report of Her Majesty's Inspectorate:

> As public interest in *managerial efficiency* and *institutional effectiveness* has increased, there has been a general acknowledgement of the need to use *performance indicators* to monitor the higher education system ... some concrete information on the extent to which the *benefits expected from educational expenditure* are actually secured ... [an] approach finding most favour in 1989 and 1990 is the classification of performance indicators within an *input, output, process model* (HMI, 1991, my italics).

In searching for indicators 'which allow institutions to assess their own *fitness for purpose*', the report suggests a range of reference points which enable an 'assessment of achievement against a defined objective': 'cost effective indicators', 'academic operations indicators' such as 'inputs' (eg, applications in relation to numbers or ratios per place), 'process' (eg, value-added) and 'output' (eg, employer satisfaction).

This changed language is not conducive to the theoretical reflection, the philosophical speculation, the sociological explaining that had provided the substance to an academically respectable course of educational studies. Rather is it the language of control – a language through which the traditional role of the universities can be, and has been, undermined.

To summarize: to predict and to influence the future depends upon an understanding of the past. In the past, universities provided an academic respectability to teaching as it strove to become a profession. That respectability was provided by a body of knowledge – from ancient philosophers to more recent sociologists – upon which the practitioners might draw. But there were always those who remained deeply suspicious of theory and of its relevance to practice. That suspicion had its philosophical base, arising from a particular doubt about the logical status of theory and of its relationship to practice. It also received political support, first, because the weak philosophical base gave rise, so it was claimed, to uncritical and damaging ideological teaching (reflected in the various kinds of child-centred approaches to teaching) and, second, because there was always a readiness to economize where savings could be made – and to do this by impoverishing the language of education.

In looking to the future, what kinds of argument are required to counter the atheoretical basis upon which the role of universities is being systematically questioned?

The Future and the Exercise of Power

In looking to the future one needs to distinguish between a future which, in the light of rational considerations, is desirable and should be argued for and a future which is likely to occur because of the exercise of power by those who have demonstrated their hostility to university involvement in teacher training. In this chapter I can do little else than argue a point while admitting that argument, even if valid (and I must leave it to others to arbitrate on that), may today be of little avail. However, it is necessary, in parenthesis as it were, to attend a little to the exercise of power.

Under the 1944 Education Act, Central Advisory Councils were established, with wide representation, which had a right to be consulted on major developments in educational policy including the training of teachers. When asked what the duties of a member of that Advisory Council were, one member was informed by the Permanent Secretary, Sir John Maude, 'to be prepared to die at the first ditch as soon as politicians get their hands on education'. The long-standing tradition of an independent body of Inspectors was maintained and enhanced, which could give impartial and professional advice to Ministers on the training of teachers as well as on all other matters, and which could, without fear, be critical of policy. The impartiality of civil servants was unquestioned as part of a tradition of public service unaffected by market forces. Power was devolved to local authorities which accepted responsibility for schools, training colleges and further education. There was a clear distinction between organizational decisions (a political matter) and professional judgement. It was, one might say, a partnership with mutual respect for the respective contribution of the different partners, a delicate balance between different interests.

No one would, I suspect, believe that the balance was exactly right or that the partnership was ideal. Where for instance were parents? Were local authorities the most appropriate bodies for supervising the aspiring higher education system of training colleges? Should not government, which paid the bill, play a more active part in determining the aims and content of the curriculum, initially in schools but then later in those university departments responsible for professional training?

Partnerships can change in answer to such questions. They can adjust. New partners can be introduced and the form of the relationships be altered without the general spirit of partnership being destroyed. None the less, what we have witnessed in the last few years is the destruction of that framework which was created or strengthened by the 1944 Act. Central Advisory Councils have been abolished, local authorities so enfeebled as to have little power, Her Majesty's Inspectorate so decimated as no longer to be able to provide the breadth of intelligence or the depth of independence which it once did. Civil servants have been moved from office for offering the impartial advice on teacher training which was once their duty to give. Advice instead has been sought from unaccountable bodies with clear political agendas and the government has taken to itself power which enables it to interfere in universities and colleges to a degree which was inconceivable only a few years ago. Furthermore, the language of control – the language of audits and performance indicators, of inputs and outputs, of quality assurance and TQM, of competences and of specific objectives – provides the means whereby that power might be exercised.

In looking to the future one might wonder whether universities can continue to provide professional training for teachers – those universities at least which are not yet beguiled by this language and which remain faithful to the aspirations of the Dean of Christ Church when he argued for university involvement. In 1895, the Dean expressed the hope that Oxford

> may send out men who will help to keep up a high standard and conception of teaching in all the sub divisions of secondary education ... who are thoroughly able to appreciate, and realise and take into their own minds and character the best gifts that Oxford ... has to offer (Bryce Report, 1895, pp.v, 204).

There was seen to be a connection between 'high standards and conception of teaching' on the one hand and on the other an appreciation of what a distinctively university education should aim at. And why not? If schools are to be centres of learning, then teachers too must be rooted in a tradition of learning, of critical enquiry, of intellectual search and of that 'conversation which takes place between the generations of mankind'. An essential element in that tradition and in that conversation is a form of intellectual questioning and enquiry which cannot be reduced to the finite list of competences ordained by politicians.

The proposed 1994 legislation, described and criticized elsewhere in this book, completes the shift of balance from a genuinely university involvement in teacher training (whatever the defects that there have been in practice) to one which, with the removal of funding from the Higher Education Funding Council and with the supreme powers accruing to the Secretary of State, is by courtesy only – and only then if it is restricted to training in classroom competences.

Such a cynical accretion and misuse of power which is antipathetic to free intellectual enquiry and research would seem to point to the declining fortunes of university involvement in teacher education. It may remain, of course, but hardly in a form that is recognizably appropriate to a university. There are the cowboy institutions which have, as Dr Jackson of Exeter College suggested they might do, collected the fees and 'scattered ... the half-fledged teachers ... to the schools'. But in such universities or colleges there is nothing distinctively *university* about the contribution made by the institution, which serves instead as a convenient administrative machine for the difficult job of distribution.

However, there are two reasons for hope and which point to a future in which there will be flourishing departments of educational studies, with a distinctive agenda worthy of universities and closely involved in the training of teachers. The first is that the government is no more likely to succeed in this policy than in its other policies. The reason for this is simple and should be obvious to anyone who has reflected on the limited capacity of the state to engage in 'utopian engineering'. That limited capacity is due to the complex nature of that which is to be organized and the limited knowledge and skills of those who have to do the organizing. Just as there is little likelihood that the centralized running of 25,000 schools will be more efficient than the local administration of, on average, 250 schools (Whitehall knows less than the town hall about Alderman Smithers Comprehensive School), so too there is little likelihood that the admission, organization, placement and assessment of 45,000 trainee teachers will be as efficiently undertaken by 25,000 schools (whether or not in consortia) as by 90 higher education institutions. Those who are familiar with teacher training, even those who are ardent advocates of reform, know the complexity of the task and the subtlety of the decisions which have to be made. There is a massive amount of tacit knowledge in the handling of difficult and often fraught situations – of adult learners in contact with reluctant school children. Such tacit knowledge by definition cannot be captured in the finite list of competences or in the regulations established by civil servants. The present Bill, if passed, will have to be later amended to cope with the unforeseen difficulties which will emerge. Part of the cause of incompetence lies in the lack of consultation – and that is a general point: unless views on complex matters are subject to open and critical scrutiny they are likely to be wrong at least in detail.

The second reason why the future of universities' involvement in teacher education should be assured is that the teachers themselves see how closely connected are their own aspirations to professional status with a university partnership in which distinctive roles of each partner are clearly recognized and respected. And that professional aspiration cannot for ever be suppressed.

However, it is important if that partnership is to provide the basis for the future commitment of universities to teacher training that the distinctive contribution of universities should be recognized – especially by the universities themselves – and the central argument is connected with the nature of teaching as a profession.

Teaching as a Profession

In understanding the future relationship of universities to the development of teaching, both through initial training and through subsequent staff development, there are three aspects of the *profession* of teaching to which I wish to draw the attention of the reader.

Knowledge

A profession has a knowledge base, an expertise, which goes beyond common sense, the acquisition of which requires systematic teaching.

There are three aspects of this knowledge base. The first is the knowledge of that which is to be taught – the kind of knowledge which is acquired in the study for one's degree in history, say, or in mathematics. The second is the knowledge of how this knowledge might be communicated in an intellectually respectable and yet accessible form to those who do not understand. The third is the ability so to reflect on experience and so to subject those reflections to critical enquiry, that the teacher will be able to form a *defensible* theoretical perspective – a view about motivation, differential abilities, interests, worthwhile subject matter – which will direct and sustain the teaching. I stress the word 'defensible' because the dogmatic clinging to a set of beliefs is not the mark of a professional. The belief must be held for reasons and, like any rationally held belief, they will adapt to contrary evidence and counter reasons.

The formation of the teacher, if he or she is to be considered a professional, must contain these three sorts of knowledge – the content of what is to be taught, the 'knowing how' of communicating it, and the cognitive tendency and capacity to grow through reflection and criticism. Teaching is a practical activity certainly, but it is one that can be engaged in more or less intelligently, more or less critically. And to be intelligent and critical requires an acquaintance with traditions of critical enquiry which have formed the views that we have.

Such traditions have two aspects – first, what we know about how (for example) the logical structure of a subject might be translated into terms which are intelligible and motivating for the young and often reluctant learner; second, how we set about questioning received and often untested methods, ways of proceeding, such that we might internalize and develop that knowledge – and, indeed, build upon it.

Universities are clearly the places where such traditions of knowledge – and thus of professional learning – take place, not only because they attract the experts in such matters but also because they embody that very tradition of critical enquiry based on knowledge which is so essential to the professional independence of the teacher. The arguments levelled against such a view are not very persuasive. There are of course those who think like Dr Sheila Lawlor (BBC, 1991), who advises the government on such matters, that theory, if needed at all, should be balanced with St Thomas Aquinas and some text from the early Christian fathers. Personally I like the suggestion. Having spent three years studying *Summa Contra Gentiles*, I am possibly the only member of a university department of education thus qualified to prepare the next generation of teachers. But I have to admit that in no way did such learning help me when I first confronted the problem of teaching in Camden Town. Somehow the children there did not share the same list of virtues as St Thomas.

Values

What distinguishes a member of a profession from the members of other occupational groups is a commitment to certain values, to certain norms of appropriate conduct, to a certain quality of relationship with those whom they are serving. Such values and norms define the nature of the relationship peculiar to that occupation. They reflect an acknowledgement of the client as someone to be served to the best of *their* interest rather than someone to be exploited to the best of one's own. Teachers are committed to those values and relationships which belong to the very special transaction which goes on between teacher and learner. Such a transaction is an introduction to a world of ideas, of aspirations, of what has been (and of what can be) achieved. The values of teaching as a profession, which professional preparation must strive to nurture, are, therefore, those that pertain to the quality of this transaction: a caring for one's subject as something of value to be shared and a caring for all pupils, irrespective of age and ability.

This particular moral formation is within the university tradition as experienced by many – the caring for a subject and how it is communicated because of its worth not of its utility, the concern for evidence and reasoned argument, the respect for alternative viewpoints if they can be defended, the search for understanding and for a theoretical grasp which helps the student to make sense of experience – in this case, the experience of schooling and education.

Such values are precious. They are hard come by. They are easily lost. How important it is to preserve institutions and then to plug into those institutions, where they are an essential (albeit endangered) element in the maintenance of those values.

Control

The third aspect of a profession lies in the authority and the control which its members are able to exercise over their own affairs – setting and maintaining standards of performance, identifying areas which require further research and development, providing expert comment and criticism. Such a professional role has long been denied teachers in England, though not in Scotland. Yet it is essentially a recognition of the fact that the kind of judgement and practice that teachers engage in cannot be encapsulated in a book of rules or in legislation. Teachers are inevitably involved in questions about goals, not simply about means to those goals. They live within a moral framework to which they contribute as much as they draw from it. This moral framework in which they have, through their responsibility for young people, a distinctive place, needs to be reflected in codes of conduct, disciplinary procedures, conditions of entry, analysis of professional needs and advice to government.

It was to support and to enhance this professional aspect of teaching that the Schools Council was established in 1964, an attempt, in the words of the great civil servant Derek Morrell (1966), 'to democratise the problem solving as we try, as best we can, to develop an educational approach appropriate to a permanent condition of change'. That democratization was led by the teachers whose professional responsibility was to find solutions to the content and methods of learning suited to the needs of those in their care. Such solutions had to address questions of value in a context where there is so little consensus on matters which are of crucial importance to society and indeed to the learners themselves. Though led by teachers, it had nevertheless to be a joint enterprise with other constituencies within the community who had a stake in the products of schooling, and with those in universities who might contribute, through research and scholarship and expert knowledge, to the search for solutions.

A partnership was envisaged which again is being resurrected, not in that form, but through a General Teaching Council which would exercise the kind of control referred to and which would again endorse the necessary partnership in the democratization of decision making.

The Future of the University Department

I have said that in looking to the future one can both predict, in the light of various political and economic forces, and argue for what should be the case. I want in this final section to conclude what, from the changes we have experienced and from the essentially professional nature of teaching, needs to be argued for in the establishment of a different though distinctive role for university departments. There are three aspects of this.

Critical tradition

It is difficult to envisage a healthy teaching profession which is not rooted in a tradition of critical enquiry. If schools are to be 'learning societies' – centres where the mind is developed, where 'intelligence is acquired', where the young come to appreciate what is worthwhile – then the teachers themselves must be part of a wider learning and critical society. They too must be able to relate to places where their own understanding and knowledge can be brought up to date and enriched. They must be able to share in a deeper argument about the values and the purposes served by education. Universities at their best are centres of such tradition, and as such they provide a much needed service to schools. Such a critical tradition is not a matter of applying theory to practice. Much more is it a matter of learning how to theorize about practice, but to do so in an informed way and in a context where questioning and 'making sense of' are activities which are unashamedly the main business.

Research

One aspect of this critical tradition is that of learning from and engaging in research – the kind of research which Morrell envisaged the Schools Council as promoting and the results of which would illuminate the decisions which teachers necessarily make. Such research may not be fundamental within the disciplines of sociology or psychology but it would draw upon them and it would systematically address the questions which teachers ask and which need answers. University departments of educational studies would be closely associated with those departments, the main purpose of which was not to illuminate educational qualities but to provide the theoretical understandings of society or of individuals of relevance to education. Certainly such a central professional body as the General Teaching Council would need to draw upon such a research tradition.

For that reason, Scotland has for 70 years established a close relationship between the Educational Institute of Scotland (EIS) representing the teachers and the Scottish Council for Research in Education. The Research Committee of the EIS, when that connection was established in 1928, exhorted its membership 'to justify our claim to professional status by showing a greater keenness in all that concerns the science and art of our profession' (Wake, 1988). Practical research into the aims, context and methods (including assessment) of education was seen as essential to teaching as a profession, requiring links with centres where that research was conducted and from where it could be disseminated through higher degrees, courses and publications.

Centres of expertise

There is a knowledge – a 'knowing that' about the translation of complex ideas into the mode of representation suited to the learner and a 'knowing how' to put it across and to reflect systematically upon one's experience – which is crucial if teaching is to be seen (as indeed it deserves to be) as something more than practical common sense. There are those, usually successful practitioners, who have the capacity to distil that knowledge and 'know-how' and to communicate it through example and critique of practice, through reference and guidance, through exhortation and exposition. The manner of telling should not detract from the expertise of the teller. If all university departments were destroyed then very shortly new centres of expertise would arise to serve the needs of schools, providing a service in such matters as subject teaching, assessment, special needs, equal opportunity and vocational training. Such expertise would be based upon knowledge, experience and research – precisely the service which universities are there to give.

The role of the university department therefore is essentially that of providing, first, a centre of expertise relevant to teaching; second, a critical tradition within which both the trainee and the experienced teacher might learn in an informed and questioning way to examine educational practice; and, third, a centre of relevant research. In the absence of these three 'services' – the distinctive jobs of a university – it is difficult to see how teaching can long maintain its claim to be a profession, a claim that must be based upon an expertise grounded in specialist knowledge, in critical enquiry and in relevant research. On the other hand, such a claim must not be understood as a defence of the status quo. There are several reasons for that.

There is no doubt that the quality and the validity of the university-based knowledge has, in many cases, been undermined by an indefensible separation of theory from practice and of universities from schools. To be intelligent about the practice of teaching requires, on the part of the university, a constant and real involvement in that practice. It requires, too, a deep respect for the understandings of the teachers and of the contribution which they make to professional training and development. Such at least was the aspiration of the Schools Council and is embodied in the proposals for the General Teaching Council.

Presently there are many attempts to create or to renew partnerships between the higher education institutions and the schools in the training and continued professional development of teachers. In many cases, these appear to be no more than last-ditch attempts of those institutions to stay alive, especially where the impoverished theory remains separate from practice and where the employees of the one remain aloof from the employees of the other. Trainees still are 'scattered to the schools' without too much thought being given to the nature and the quality of that experience. The university or college lecturers too often remain as strangers to the practices they are theorizing about and preparing the trainees for. Therefore, a lot needs to change. But it is not easy. How can one be both academically respectable and professionally relevant?

Moreover it is difficult to see how, even in terms of theory and research alone, there can be the quality which warrants so many places set apart for that purpose. There is a limit to the number of people who can maintain and enhance that research tradition which should inform practice and which is the hallmark of a university. There are two conclusions, therefore, which I would wish to draw.

First, in a few years' time, there will be a much reduced number of departments of educational studies in universities – possibly no more than 30 which have a tradition of research, scholarship and critical enquiry serving the profession of teaching. Such centres might well have their satellite institutions to make easier the access from schools.

Second, the greater responsibility of schools for initiating new recruits into teaching will be both recognized and institutionalized, possibly under the leadership and guidance of a General Teaching Council, certainly in cooperation with the more limited number of university centres of research, scholarship and enquiry. It will take seriously the advocacy of Morrell (1966):

> Jointly, we need to define the characteristics of change – relying, whenever possible, on objective data rather than on opinions unsupported by evidence. Jointly, we need to sponsor the research and development work necessary to respond to change. Jointly, we must evaluate the results of such work, using both judgement and measurement techniques .... Jointly, we need to recognise that freedom and order can no longer be reconciled through implicit acceptance of a broadly ranging and essentially static consensus on educational aims and methods.

The future, then, lies in the success or otherwise of the joint enterprise. Neither past arrangements (with several glorious exceptions) nor present government proposals have it right. But 'rightness' must rest partly in recognizing the distinctive aims of the university and how those aims might be partnered with the professional expertise of the teachers in the preparation of the next generation of teachers.

References

BBC (1991) 'File on Four', 19 February.
Bryce Report (1895) *Royal Commission on Secondary Education*, London: HMSO.
Her Majesty's Inspectorate (1991) *Higher Education in the Polytechnics and Colleges*, London: HMSO.
Morrell, D (1966) *Education and Change*, Lecture I, The Annual Joseph Payne Memorial Lectures, London: College of Preceptors.
O'Connor, D J (1957) *Introduction to the Philosophy of Education*, Routledge and Kegan Paul: London.
Wake, R (1988) 'Research as the hallmark of the professional: Scottish teachers and research in the early 1920s', *Scottish Educational Review*, 20, 1.

Index